Medical Sciences at a Glance: Practice Workbook

This title is also available as an e-book.
For more details, please see
www.wiley.com/buy/9780470654491
or scan this QR code:

Medical Sciences at a Glance: Practice Workbook

Jakub Scaber BMBCh BA (Hons) MRCP

MRC/MND Association Clinical Research Fellow
Nuffield Department of Clinical Neurosciences
University of Oxford
Oxford, UK

Lecturer, St Anne's College
University of Oxford
Oxford, UK

Faisal Rahman BMBCh BA (Hons) MA (Oxon)

Internal Medicine Resident
Boston Medical Center
Boston, MA, USA

Peter Abrahams FRCS FRCR DO(Hon) FHEA

Professor of Clinical Anatomy
Warwick Medical School
Warwick, UK

Professor of Clinical Anatomy
Examiner for the FRCS and MRCS
St George's University
Grenada, West Indies

WILEY Blackwell

Library of Congress Cataloging-in-Publication Data is available

A catalogue record for this book is available from the British Library.

Cover image: iStock © Dra_schwartz
Cover design by Meaden Creative

Set in 9/11.5pt Times New Roman by SPi Publisher Services, Pondicherry, India
Printed and bound in Malaysia by Vivar Printing Sdn Bhd

1   2014

Contents

Preface

Examinations often have an overexposed role in our learning process. Preclinical medical examinations are no different: the sheer volume of detail in a range of subjects that covers seemingly theoretical and dry concepts makes many students wonder why they chose to read medicine.

At that stage the syllabus appears vast. Textbooks go into too much detail for the revision. Past examination papers may be available without answers. Increasingly, universities have question databases that they protect from students and their ability to share them instantaneously. Currently available published study materials are focused on membership examinations and finals, and few go into any depth explaining answers.

In this book we wanted to address these points. We know from experience that ultimately a core of facts, concepts and misunderstandings gets tested over and over again as you progress through your medical career. We have included as many of these 'pearls' as possible and provided each with a detailed answer, which will explain both the correct choice and the common pitfalls.

We strongly believe that the basic sciences are not just a group of facts to pass and to forget, but that they have real clinical applications. Although knowledge of clinical medicine and history taking is not required for this book, we have included small vignettes to bring concepts to life and to stimulate thought about the clinical relevance of each question.

When writing this book, we were aware that medical sciences are taught in very different styles across the UK and elsewhere. We could not create a book that would be ideal for everyone and chose a subdivision by subject. We included a mix of question types to cater for different approaches and to provide variety to better test your knowledge. Questions are arranged in exam-like chapters each containing 15 multiple-choice questions, five extended matching questions, five true/false questions and five short answer questions.

We hope that you find this book stimulating and rewarding in your revision for your examinations and beyond.

Jakub Scaber
Oxford

Faisal Rahman
Boston

Peter Abrahams
Warwick

Acknowledgements

There are a number of people without whom this book would not have been possible.

We would like to thank our chapter reviewers who provided guidance and expert input: Professor Leo Dasso (Biochemistry and Pharmacology) and Dr Dirk Bäumer (Neuroscience). We are grateful to those colleagues who kindly provided images (as attributed) and to Professor Michael Hortsch who went to great lengths to make available slides from the University of Michigan database.

We thank the entire editorial team at Wiley-Blackwell, especially Elizabeth Johnston, Laura Murphy, Helen Harvey and Katrina Rimmer, for their unwavering support for this project.

JS would like to thank his wife Agnieszka for her encouragement and patience for many months. JS is also grateful to Dr John Goodfellow for his support. Without him this book would not have taken off.

Introduction: an approach to answering questions

The most important advice that can be repeated again and again is of course to read the question thoroughly first and then read the answer. This obvious point is the most common reason for getting answers wrong: it means what it says so don't skip to the end of the question because you get bored and don't read the answer first – you will fall for the traps. The question may sometimes seem irrelevant but more often than not it contains important clues that are either essential or very helpful in answering the question.

Multiple-choice questions (MCQ)

Multiple-choice questions remain one of the most commonly used examination tools. They are relatively easy to write and allow for computerised marking and analysis of replies using a variety of statistical methods. Most nationwide examination schemes such as a number of Royal College membership examinations and the US medical licensing examinations (USMLEs) use these.

Downsides of this question type are that they can be geared towards testing of facts rather than concepts, and can sometimes invite students to guess the answer which seems most sensible. Examiners try to overcome this by creating questions that will require you to integrate multiple facts and by inserting distractors (obvious mistakes).

Classical MCQs (closed questions)

These questions ask a specific point of information; they are closed. If you know the answer you can answer the question even without knowing the five options, and should try and do this during exam conditions. It allows you to bypass answers that have been put in to distract you. If you struggle to do this, look at the answers and try to eliminate the obvious false answers and pick from the remaining ones.

Best-of-five questions (open questions)

You will be presented with an open-ended question, such as 'what is a difference between A and B?' or 'what is the most likely cause for this?'. Reading the question thoroughly remains key when answering these questions; you should have a fair idea about what potential answers you are looking for. You will then have to look at each answer in turn and decide individually if (a), (b), (c), etc. are true and then pick from the ones you have decided to be the most likely answers (hopefully only one).

A special type of open-ended MCQ is that written like a 'true/false' question, with multiple statements. They are becoming less popular and are the only MCQs where it is permissible to read the answers before reading the questions. Because they are still in use, we have included a few of these examples which will be preceded by a statement like 'Which *one* of the following statements is true?'.

True/False questions

These are supposed to be the easiest questions to write and are often sentences that could be taken out of a textbook, some of which have been modified to incorporate common mistakes in understanding by students.

Because they can be regarded as easy on their own, examiners will try to increase their difficulty. For example, two or more pieces of information can be included in each statement, of which only one is false. Sometimes negative marking is used to increase the perceived difficulty (see below).

True/False questions are obviously centred around the statements – and these have to be read carefully. True/False questions are the only questions where you may choose to start the question by reading these statements, but do not discard the question stem entirely as it may contain vital clues which may help you in judging whether the statements are true or not.

Extended matching questions (EMQs)

An increasingly popular way to ask questions that overcomes some of the predictability of MCQs. For a given set of answers, there are usually a number of direct questions, five in the case of this book.

Again, the best way is to think of the answer to the question first and then find it on the list. If you know the answer, you will find it or an answer that is closely related. The list will usually be sufficiently long and the timing of the question sufficiently brief to not allow analysing every answer to find the best one for the particular question.

If you cannot find the answer after a quick scroll through the ones available, you may wish to mark the question as unfinished and move on. The worst mistake you can make with EMQs is to ponder over the options available while time for your remaining questions is passing.

Short answer questions (SAQs)

A very good question style that used to allow for a variety of question types such as: lists, fill in the gaps, analyse the data, etc. However, it has fallen out of favour since the advent of electronic marking: SAQs still have to be marked by hand. This question style also allows some interpretation of the questions by both examinee and examiner and thus introduces an element of subjectivity.

The key to answering these questions is to know how many points can be gained from the question. It's usually five in our book so aim to list five facts or to make five key points. Trying to list more or write more will usually irritate the examiner who will have to pick the five relevant ones. You may be marked down for superfluous information or, worse, for the mistakes you have made in the additional information provided.

Positive and negative marking

We believe that this issue usually creates unnecessary anxiety amongst students. Positive marking is standard currently – you get a mark for a correct answer and no points for either a wrong or an absent answer. What follows from this is that an absent answer is a wasted opportunity. Because you do not get punished for guessing, you should never leave a single question blank even if you have no clue: you get a 50% chance of scoring in True/False questions, 20% in MCQs and usually <10% in EMQs.

Negative marking introduces a negative mark for a wrong answer. Because your results are usually analysed against your peers, this means that the pass mark usually falls drastically when this marking scheme is introduced. However, don't be tempted to leave too many questions blank – you don't score for blank questions. The approach to negative marking depends on the question type.

- **True/False**: these questions are more likely to be marked negatively. Using positive marking, even a monkey trained for the task will score 50% on these questions and a score of 70% means that you actually only got 40% right and guessed the rest. A score of 50% on negative marking means that you probably knew about half the syllabus with certainty. If you do a True/False paper with negative marking, the key question is what to do with statements where you don't know or aren't sure. You can either leave them blank or answer them, risking a negative mark. How you deal with this will be individual: some people do very well by guessing, while others will fall for the hidden traps time and time again. If you are a person who second guesses and analyses questions a lot, you will probably find yourself in the group of people who don't guess well. The best way to find out, however, is to do a number of past papers yourself using negative marking and see which strategy gives you more points (statistically both should be equally effective).

- **MCQs and EMQs**: rarely negatively marked. Guessing these questions with negative marking makes absolutely no statistical sense unless you can exclude all but two answers. Even then, not answering the question is probably better, but again try the method suggested in the previous point.

- **SAQs**: these questions have always been negatively marked in a way as false information results in a penalty, though overall the lowest mark is usually 0.

Using hints other than knowledge to answer questions

This is not an uncommon trick advised by some students and found on the internet. We would recommend you avoid these techniques, which are known to people who write questions. A non-exhaustive list of such bad advice includes the following.

- 'Questions that contain always/never are generally false.' (Unfortunately we still see some use of these questions which can be misleading and invite second guessing of the meaning of the question.)

- Using grammar or syntax to guess the answer, e.g. picking the only past tense answer for a past tense question.

- Analysing answers and deducing the most common combination, e.g. in a two-word answer, picking the answer which has the most common first word and the most common second word.

Related titles

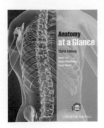

Anatomy at a Glance, 3rd edition
Omar Faiz, Simon Blackburn and David
Moffat
www.wiley.com/buy/9781444336092

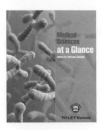

Medical Sciences at a Glance
Michael D. Randall
www.wiley.com/buy/9781118360927

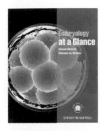

Embryology at a Glance
Samuel Webster and Rhiannon de Wreede
www.wiley.com/buy/9780470654538

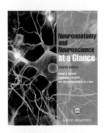

Neuroanatomy and Neuroscience at a Glance,
4th edition
Roger A. Barker and Francesca Cicchetti
www.wiley.com/buy/9780470657683

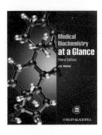

Medical Biochemistry at a Glance, 3rd edition
J. G. Salway
www.wiley.com/buy/9780470654514

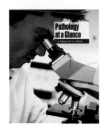

Pathology at a Glance
Caroline Finlayson and Barry Newell
www.wiley.com/buy/9781405136501

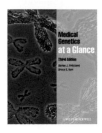

Medical Genetics at a Glance, 3rd edition
Dorian J. Pritchard and Bruce R. Korf
www.wiley.com/buy/9780470656549

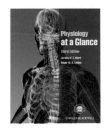

Physiology at a Glance, 3rd edition
Jeremy P.T. Ward and Roger W.A. Linden
www.wiley.com/buy/9780470659786

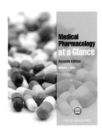

Medical Pharmacology at a Glance, 7th edition
Michael J. Neal
www.wiley.com/buy/9780470657898

How to use your textbook

Features contained within your textbook

This textbook contains 12 separate examinations divided by 6 subject areas. Each exam contains 15 multiple-choice questions (MCQs), five extended matching questions (EMQs), five True/False questions and five short answer questions (SAQs). The answers appear at the end of each exam.

Each chapter can be done as a timed examination and should not take longer than 60–90 minutes.

If you would like to score your examination we suggest the following weighting:
- MCQs: 2 points per question
- EMQs: 5 points per question
- True/False: 5 points per question
- SAQ: points suggested in question (usually 5 points).

The best time to use this book is towards the end of lecture courses but early in your revision – you will benefit most if you study the questions together with the answers; this includes both wrong answers and answers you were not sure about.

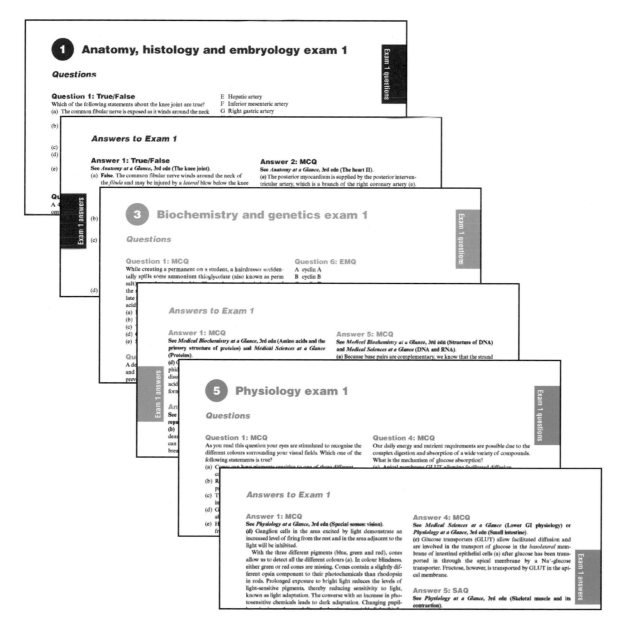

The anytime, anywhere textbook

Wiley E-Text

Your book is also available to purchase as a **Wiley E-Text: Powered by VitalSource** version – a digital, interactive version of this book which you own as soon as you download it.

Your **Wiley E-Text** allows you to:

- **Search**: Save time by finding terms and topics instantly in your book, your notes, even your whole library (once you've downloaded more textbooks)
- **Note and Highlight**: Colour code, highlight and make digital notes right in the text so you can find them quickly and easily
- **Organise**: Keep books, notes and class materials organised in folders inside the application
- **Share**: Exchange notes and highlights with friends, classmates and study groups
- **Upgrade**: Your textbook can be transferred when you need to change or upgrade computers.

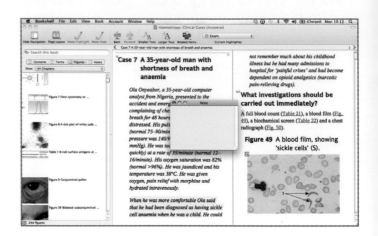

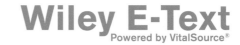

The **Wiley E-Text** version will also allow you to copy and paste any photograph or illustration into assignments, presentations and your own notes.

To access your Wiley E-Text:

- Visit **www.vitalsource.com/software/bookshelf/downloads** to download the bookshelf application to your computer, laptop, tablet or mobile device.
- Open the bookshelf application on your computer and register for an account.
- Follow the registration process.

The VitalSource Bookshelf can now be used to view your Wiley E-Text **on iOS, Android and Kindle Fire!**

- **For iOS**: Visit the app store to download the VitalSource Bookshelf: **http://bit.ly/17ib3XS**
- **For Android**: Visit the Google Play Market to download the VitalSource Bookshelf: **http://bit.ly/ZMEGvo**
- **For Kindle Fire, Kindle Fire 2 or Kindle Fire HD**: Simply install the VitalSource Bookshelf onto your Fire (see how at **http://bit.ly/11BVFn9**). You can now sign in with the email address and password you used when you created your VitalSource Bookshelf Account.

Full E-Text support for mobile devices is available at: **http://support.vitalsource.com**

CourseSmart

CourseSmart gives you instant access (via computer or mobile device) to this Wiley-Blackwell e-book and its extra electronic functionality, at 40% off the recommended retail print price. See all the benefits at: **www.coursesmart.com/students**

Instructors … receive your own digital desk copies!

CourseSmart also offers instructors an immediate, efficient, and environmentally friendly way to review this book for your course. For more information visit **www.coursesmart.com/instructors.**

With CourseSmart, you can create lecture notes quickly with copy and paste, and share pages and notes with your students. Access your **CourseSmart** digital book from your computer or mobile device instantly for evaluation, class preparation, and as a teaching tool in the classroom.

Simply sign in at **http://instructors.coursesmart.com/bookshelf** to download your Bookshelf and get started. To request your desk copy, hit 'Request Online Copy' on your search results or book product page.

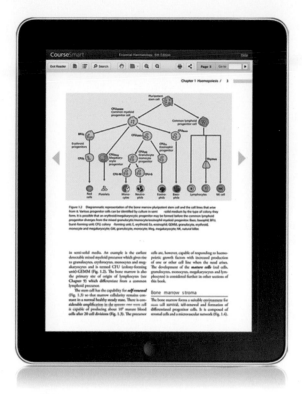

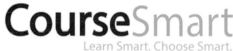

We hope you enjoy using your new book. Good luck with your studies!

Questions

Question 1: True/False
Which of the following statements about the knee joint are true?
(a) The common fibular nerve is exposed as it winds around the neck of the tibia and may be injured by a medial blow to the knee.
(b) A lateral blow to the knee may cause injury to the medial collateral ligament, the medial meniscus and the anterior cruciate ligament, also known as the 'terrible triad'.
(c) The patella usually dislocates medially.
(d) The knee joint is a complex as well as a compound synovial hinge joint.
(e) A disc herniation at L4–L5 that compresses the exiting spinal nerve may result in ipsilateral wasting of the extensors of the knee joint.

Question 2: MCQ
A 45-year-old publican comes to the emergency department with central crushing chest pain that suddenly began 90 minutes ago. An ECG indicates injury of the posterior aspects of the septum and left ventricle. Which of the following arteries is most likely occluded?
(a) Anterior interventricular artery
(b) Right marginal artery
(c) Left circumflex artery
(d) SA-nodal artery
(e) Right coronary artery

Question 3: SAQ (5 points)
Describe how knowledge of the anatomy of the facial nerve could help you localise the level of the lesion in a person with a drooped left face. What signs and symptoms other than weakness may help you localise the lesion?

Question 4: MCQ
Skin cancers are responsible for around one-third of all human malignancies, and basal cell carcinomas are the most common skin cancer. Which skin layer do basal cell carcinomas arise from (Figure 1.1)?

Question 5: MCQ
During a classic embryology experiment, ectodermal cells are taken from the ectoderm of an embryo. In a neutral medium, they develop into the epidermal layer of skin. This is an example which is best described by which of the following terms?
(a) Fate
(b) Specification
(c) Determination
(d) Differentiation
(e) Commitment

Question 6: EMQ
A Left gastroepiploic artery
B Right gastroepiploic artery
C Celiac trunk
D Left gastric artery
E Hepatic artery
F Inferior mesenteric artery
G Right gastric artery
H Superior mesenteric artery
I Gastroduodenal artery
J Splenic artery
K Pudendal artery

For each of the scenarios below, choose the most appropriate answer from the list above.
(1) Which artery is compressible during a laparotomy as it travels through the free border of the lesser omentum?
(2) A 26-year-old woman comes in with a history of nausea and vomiting and is admitted to the emergency department. She has had a surgical correction of her scoliosis 2 months ago. An urgent barium meal shows almost total obstruction of the third part of the duodenum. Which blood vessel has probably caused the obstruction?
(3) A 53-year-old accountant is admitted to the emergency department with severe epigastric pain and haematemesis. He is haemodynamically unstable and is rushed for laparotomy. The surgeon finds profuse bleeding from a perforated ulcer in the posterior wall of the first segment of the duodenum. Which artery is most probably injured?
(4) A 78-year-old woman comes to see you with a lump on her back end. On examination, you find a 1 cm irregular mass on the anterior wall of the anal canal. Biopsy reveals an adenocarcinoma. Which artery does the tumour receive its blood supply from?
(5) A 36-year-old publican comes to the emergency department after he vomited blood earlier this morning. He is

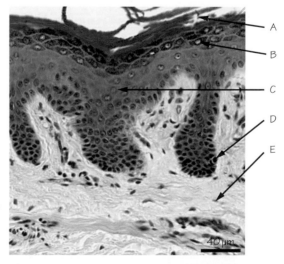

Figure 1.1 Skin layers. Reproduced with permission from Peckham M (2011) *Histology at a Glance*. Oxford: Wiley-Blackwell.

haemodynamically stable and an upper endoscopy confirms a Mallory–Weiss tear in the lower third of the oesophagus. From which artery's territory did the bleeding arise?

Question 7: SAQ (5 points)

A 40-year-old woman presents with shoulder pain. An investigation is carried out, and Figure 1.2 shows the image of her shoulder that is obtained.

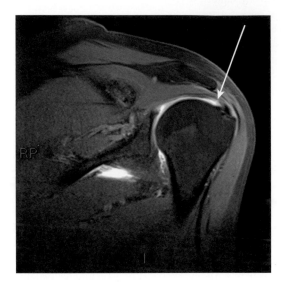

Figure 1.2 Image of the shoulder.

What imaging technique was used and what are its advantages and disadvantages? Which anatomical structure is affected by pathology (see arrow)?

Question 8: MCQ

A 56-year-old man presents with progressively worsening medial foot pain and walking difficulties. He is unable to plantarflex his great toe on the right, but able to plantarflex the remaining toes. What problem is underlying the pain and weakness?
(a) Deep fibular neuropathy
(b) Flexor hallucis longus tendinopathy
(c) L5 spinal neuropathy
(d) Tibial neuropathy
(e) First metatarsal fracture

Question 9: MCQ

A 44-year-old man presents with a vesicular rash in the distribution of T3 on the right. He complains of burning pain, particularly on his back. What is the innervation of the back skin in that distribution?
(a) Anterior ramus of T3
(b) Anterior roots of T3
(c) Posterior ramus of T3
(d) Third intercostal nerve
(e) Long thoracic nerve

Question 10: SAQ (5 points)

A 40-year-old man presents with severe loin pain that he cannot get comfortable with. He is suspected to have kidney stone disease in the ureters, and so he is given intravenous morphine and an investigation is arranged, the results of which are shown in Figure 1.3.

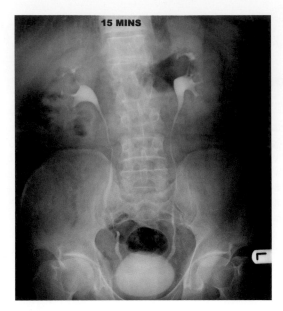

Figure 1.3 Results from investigation.

What is the name of this imaging technique and what are the two ways it can be obtained? On the image, mark the three spots where a kidney stone is most likely to lodge.

Question 11: True/False

A 7-year-old child comes in with a sore throat and difficulty breathing through his nose; he has a history of recurrent middle ear infections. These symptoms arise from enlargement of lymphatic tissue collectively known as Waldeyer's ring. Which of the following are parts of this ring protecting the respiratory tract?
(a) Nasopharyngeal lymphatics
(b) Submental lymphatics
(c) Lingual lymphatics
(d) Submandibular lymphatics
(e) Tubular lymphatics

Question 12: EMQ

A Ectoderm
B Endoderm
C Intermediate mesoderm
D Neural crest
E Mesenchyme
F Somatic mesoderm
G Somitic mesoderm
H Splanchnic mesoderm
I Yolk sac

For each of the scenarios choose the most appropriate answer from the list above.
(1) A 55-year-old alcoholic presents with a dermatomal rash at the level of T4 on the right. It is very painful. What is the embryonic origin of the layer that provides pain sensation?
(2) An infant with a known cardiac defect is diagnosed with CHARGE syndrome, which encompasses heart defects and craniofacial abnormalities including coloboma of the eye, choanal atresia, ear abnormalities and hearing loss. The infant also develops retarded growth and development and

has genital and urinary anomalies. The development of which of the above tissue groups has most probably been impaired?

(3) A leukaemia researcher investigates the embryonic origin of lymphocytes. Apart from an initial extraembryonic origin of haematopoiesis, there is another group of haematopoietic stem cells, which arises from which intraembryonic tissue?

(4) The enteric and autonomic nervous systems are derived from neural crest cells. Before being able to adopt their varied fates, neural crest cells will need to transform into what kind of tissue?

(5) A child is born with congenital absence of the biceps. What is the embryonic origin of this muscle?

Question 13: MCQ

A 45-year-old man is found to have a new systolic murmur and is investigated with an echocardiogram (Figure 1.4). On examination and previous X-ray imaging, his heart is a normal size.

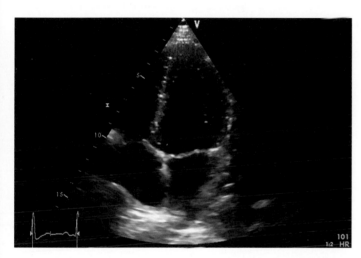

Figure 1.4 Echocardiogram showing a four-chamber view of the heart. Reproduced courtesy of Dr Richard Dobson.

Where does the ultrasound probe sit at this time point?
(a) Fifth intercostal space, midaxillary line
(b) Fifth intercostal space, midclavicular line
(c) Second intercostal space, to the left of the sternum
(d) Second intercostal space, to the right of the sternum
(e) Xiphoid process

Question 14: MCQ

A man presents with weakness and pain in his hand and forearm. On examination, he has weakness of flexion of the index and middle fingers and the distal phalanx of the thumb, altered sensation over the thenar eminence and pain that worsens on pronation. The affected nerve runs through the two bellies of the most proximal muscle it supplies and has probably been compressed by this muscle. What is the name of this muscle?
(a) Brachioradialis
(b) Flexor carpi ulnaris
(c) Flexor retinaculum of the biceps
(d) Pronator teres
(e) Supinator

Question 15: MCQ

A patient presents with haematuria and abdominal pain of 3 months duration. MRI scanning identifies a mass in the left kidney. He is scheduled for radical nephrectomy. Which of the following layers will allow the surgeon to easily separate the kidney without removing the adrenal gland?
(a) Paranephric fat
(b) Perinephric fat
(c) Peritoneum
(d) Renal (true) capsule
(e) Renal (Grota's) fascia

Question 16: EMQ

Figure 1.5 shows a CT of the thorax. Please select the letters that match the descriptions below.

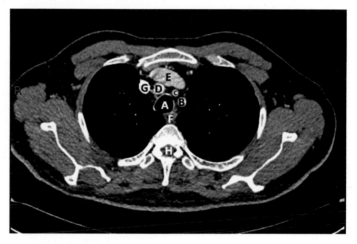

Figure 1.5 CT thorax.

(1) The thoracic duct inserts into this structure.
(2) This structure pierces the diaphragm at the level of T10.
(3) This structure has a wall made of incomplete cartilaginous rings.
(4) This structure is derived from the third branchial arch.
(5) This structure terminates at the level of L1–L2.

Question 17: True/False

Which of the following statements about groin anatomy are true?
(a) When examining for hernias, an indirect inguinal hernia will be found inferior and lateral to the pubic tubercle.
(b) During surgery for inguinal hernias, the iliohypogastric nerve may be injured, resulting in anaesthesia or chronic pain in the groin.
(c) Venepuncture of the femoral vein is achieved by inserting the needle medially to the midinguinal point.
(d) The deep inguinal ring is found lateral to the inferior epigastric artery.
(e) The internal spermatic fascia is continuous with the aponeurosis of the transversus abdominis.

Question 18: MCQ

A light microscopic image of bone (Figure 1.6) shows the following structure.

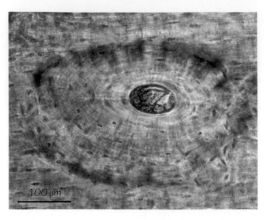

Figure 1.6 Light microscopic image of bone. Reproduced with permission from Peckham M (2011) *Histology at a Glance*. Oxford: Wiley-Blackwell

What type of bone does the section originate from?
(a) Hyaline cartilage
(b) Woven bone
(c) Cancellous bone
(d) Compact bone
(e) Cancellous or compact bone

Question 19: MCQ
A 25-year-old man is diagnosed with CNS sarcoidosis and has multiple cranial nerve defects. The treating doctor decides to test the gag reflex. Which cranial nerve lesion will produce an absent gag reflex on the affected side?
(a) IX only
(b) IX and X
(c) IX or X
(d) V_3 and X
(e) V_3 or X

Question 20: SAQ (5 points)
Describe the anatomy and clinical significance of the acetabulum.

Question 21: EMQ
A Median nerve at the wrist
B Median nerve at the elbow
C Long thoracic nerve
D C5 and C6
E C8 and T1
F Axillary nerve
G Radial nerve below the elbow
H Radial nerve above the elbow
I Ulnar nerve at the elbow
J Ulnar nerve at the wrist

For each scenario below, choose the nerve injury from the list above.
(1) A 34-year-old woman with rheumatoid arthritis comes to see you because she has felt pain in her hand and has had difficulty writing. Examination reveals pain on the lateral surface of the palm and the lateral 3½ digits, as well as the inability to maintain the middle finger and thumb opposed against resistance.
(2) A 20-year-old university student presents to your clinic because he woke up today with a left 'floppy hand'. He also complains of a headache. He was fine until yesterday, when he went to a party, at which he fell asleep slumped in a chair. Examination reveals a young man smelling of alcohol without any bruises or cuts. In the left arm there is 2/5 weakness of both wrist and finger extension and 4/5 weakness of elbow extension. Sensory testing reveals reduced sensation on the medial side of the dorsum of the wrist.
(3) You are asked to see a 71-year-old lady who has been in hospital following a cardiac valve operation, from which she has been recovering well. However, she noticed some tingling in her right hand today. On examination, you detect weakness of ad- and abduction of the fingers. In addition, she cannot flex the distal interphalangeal joints of the little and ring finger. On sensory testing, you find reduced sensation on the medial side of the right ring finger compared to its lateral side.
(4) An elderly gentleman comes into your practice for a check-up. You notice that his left arm hangs flaccidly, internally rotated at the shoulder and extended at the elbow. His forearm is pronated. He explains that his left arm became paralysed following a motorcycle injury 20 years ago.
(5) A 58-year-old woman comes for her follow-up visit 4 weeks after her breast surgery. She complains of not being able to comb her hair or store things on shelves or cupboards above her shoulder. Examination shows winging of the scapula when she pushes her hands against the wall.

Question 22: MCQ
An 85-year-old lady with known congestive cardiac failure presents with swallowing difficulty. She has a heart murmur and investigations show that a particular structure is enlarged and presses against the oesophagus. Enlargement of which structure will probably result in compression of the oesophagus?
(a) Left ventricle
(b) Left atrium
(c) Left atrial appendage
(d) Thymus
(e) Right ventricle

Question 23: True/False
Which of the following statements about early embryology are true?
(a) A 20-year-old man attends a fertility clinic and is found to have inverted organ positions and is diagnosed with Kartagener syndrome. This arises from a defect in left–right asymmetry, which is established at the primitive node by ciliary movements.
(b) During implantation, the embryonic trophoblast induces the decidual reaction, which induces maternal tissue to form the syncytiotrophoblast, which acts as an immunological and physical barrier between the maternal and fetal circulations.
(c) A woman undergoes amniocentesis after her triple test has returned with a high probability of Down syndrome. The amniotic cavity is formed during early development with splitting of the extraembryonic mesoderm into two layers.
(d) After formation of the placenta, fetal tissues are in direct contact with maternal blood in humans.

(e) With the formation of the trilaminar embryo through gastrulation in week 3, these three layers account for all embryonic tissues.

Question 24: MCQ

A 56-year-old golfer presents with intense pain on the palmar aspect of his hand that started when he was playing golf and accidentally hit the ground instead of the ball. He has not been able to straighten his medial two fingers since. On examination, his proximal palm is very tender and he has marked weakness of extension of the two medial metacarpophalangeal joints and he cannot ab- or adduct his fingers. An X-ray shows a fracture in one of the carpal bones.

(a) Capitate
(b) Hamate
(c) Scaphoid
(d) Trapezium
(e) Trapezoid

Question 25: MCQ

A 30-week pregnant woman comes to your office concerned that she is experiencing an incessant pulling sensation 'down below'. Examination localises the pulling to the labia majora. You reassure her that this is the result of a normal anatomical connection. What is the name of this connection?

(a) Suspensory ligament
(b) Broad ligament
(c) Processus vaginalis
(d) Transverse cervical (cardinal) ligament
(e) Round ligament

Question 26: EMQ

Figure 1.7 is a light micrograph of an epiphyseal growth plate.

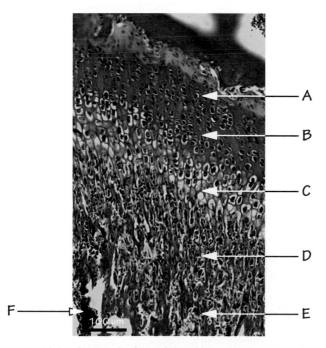

Figure 1.7 Light micrograph of an epiphyseal growth plate. Reproduced with permission from Peckham M (2011) *Histology at a Glance*. Oxford: Wiley-Blackwell.

(1) A runner prepares for a marathon and his muscle mass increases as he progresses through his training programme. Which area at the growth plate resembles this process?
(2) Neoplastic processes are characterised by multiple mitoses, but it is important to recognise that some areas will have increased mitosis in the absence of neoplasia. Which area of the normal epiphyseal plate is replicating fastest?
(3) Apoptosis is an important process that controls proliferation and tissue structure. Which area in the micrograph above is characterised by apoptosis?
(4) A patient with renal failure receives an injection of erythropoietin. Which area will this hormone act on?
(5) Where would you expect to see an osteoblastoma (tumours that arise from osteoblasts)?

Question 27: MCQ

A 17-year-old college student is brought in by ambulance unconscious. He was playing cricket without a helmet and was hit by the bat on the side of his head. A CT scan of his head shows a fracture at the junction of the parietal, occipital, frontal and sphenoid bones. Which cranial foramen does the most likely damaged structure pass through?

(a) Foramen spinosum
(b) Internal acoustic meatus
(c) Foramen ovale
(d) Foramen lacerum
(e) Superior orbital fissure

Question 28: SAQ (5 points)

Why is the diaphragm innervated by C3–5?

Question 29: MCQ

A 10-year-old obese child presents to the orthopaedic surgeons with knee pain and a detailed clinical examination reveals that the pain is referred to the knee from the hip. The child is diagnosed with a slipped femoral epiphysis. Which law describes the basis of referred pain to other joints?

(a) Bell–Magendie law
(b) Courvoisier's law
(c) Gerhardt's law
(d) Hilton's law
(e) Sherrington's law

Question 30: True/False

A 65-year-old woman with advanced breast cancer undergoes a CT of the head, chest, abdomen and pelvis to look for metastases. Which routes of spread are possible in breast cancer?

(a) Spread to thoracic vertebrae due to communications of the intercostal veins and the vertebral venous plexus.
(b) Spread to the liver via the portal vein.
(c) Spread to the brain via the vertebral venous plexus.
(d) Spread to the opposite breast through lymphatics crossing the midline.
(e) Spread to the ipsilateral supraclavicular lymph nodes is the most likely route of lymphatic spread.

Answers to Exam 1

Answer 1: True/False

See *Anatomy at a Glance*, 3rd edn (The knee joint).

(a) **False**. The common fibular nerve winds around the neck of the *fibula* and may be injured by a *lateral* blow below the knee as it is compressible against bone in that area. The common fibular nerve supplies the anterior and fibular muscle compartments of the thigh which are involved in dorsiflexion and eversion. Lack of dorsiflexion results in foot drop.

(b) **True**. Concomitant damage to both the medial collateral ligament and the medial meniscus is common because they are strongly fixed to each other.

(c) **False**. The most common direction of patellar dislocation is *laterally*. It occurs most frequently in teenagers as a result of sports injury. The quadriceps femoris pulls the patella laterally and superiorly. In healthy individuals the patella is held in place by the prominent lateral femoral condyle, a strong vastus medialis inserting medially as well as the patellofemoral ligament.

(d) **True**. The knee is a synovial joint with the following properties. First, it is compound, i.e. three or more bones contribute articular surfaces. These are the femur, tibia and patella, but *not the fibula*. Second, the knee joint is complex – it has intra-articular cartilaginous menisci, helping to make the non-matching articular surfaces congruent (matching).

(e) **False**. The extensors of the knee joint are the quadriceps femoris muscles. They are supplied by the femoral nerve which receives input from L2, L3 and L4. The nerve root exiting between the L4–L5 vertebrae is the L4 spinal nerve. However, as it exits above the compression, it is not the nerve root that is affected by disc compression at this level. An L4–L5 disc bulge instead 'catches' the L5 nerve root which is getting ready to exit in the L5–S1 vertebral foramen. Since L5 nerves do not contribute to femoral nerve innervation, no trophic changes occur in the anterior thigh.

Answer 2: MCQ

See *Anatomy at a Glance*, 3rd edn (The heart II).

(e) The posterior myocardium is supplied by the posterior interventricular artery, which is a branch of the right coronary artery (e). The right marginal artery supplies part of the right ventricle. The SA nodal artery supplies the SA node and right atrium, and is supplied by the right coronary artery in 60% of humans and by the left circumflex in 40%. The left circumflex supplies part of the left ventricle and left atrium. The left interventricular artery, the other main branch of the left coronary, supplies the anterior part of the left and right ventricles (Figure 1.8).

Answer 3: SAQ

See *Anatomy at a Glance*, 3rd edn (Cranial nerves VI–XII).

All lesions of the facial nerve result in facial droop on the ipsilateral side, but depending on the level of the injury, additional functions of the facial nerve may be affected. Thus a lesion of only the muscles of facial expression suggests a distal lesion within the parotid gland (1). A lesion at the stylomastoid foramen will additionally result in paralysis of the stylohyoid and the posterior belly of digastrics (2, impossible to assess clinically). A lesion in the facial canal will additionally result in decreased salivation and loss of taste on the anterior two-thirds of the tongue due to loss of the chorda tympani (3). It may also cause hyperacusis, hypersensitivity in hearing, due to loss of the nerve to stapedius, which exits just proximally to the chorda tympani (4). Finally, a lesion proximal to the geniculate ganglion will also cause loss of lacrimation on the affected side, as preganglionic parasympathetics branch off at the geniculate ganglion (5). Bonus: a lesion of the corticospinal tract will cause a motor deficit on the contralateral side but spare the forehead as that is innervated bilaterally by both motor cortices (6).

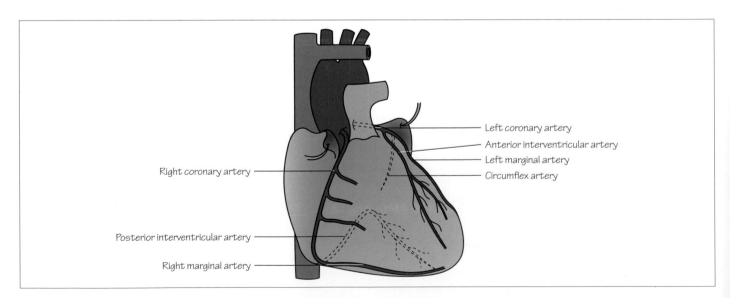

Figure 1.8 Coronary arteries. Reproduced with permission from Abrahams PH, Craven JL and Lumley JSP (2005) *Illustrated Clinical Anatomy*. London: Hodder Arnold.

Answer 4: to Exam 1 MCQ

(d) The strata of skin from outside to inside are stratum corneum (a), stratum lucidum, stratum granulosum (b), stratum spinosum (c), stratum basale (d) and the dermis (e). The stratum basale is a single layer of basophilic cells on the basement membrane that are stem cells for keratinocytes. Basal cell carcinomas arise from this layer, whereas squamous cell carcinomas arise from the stratum spinosum.

Answer 5: MCQ

(b) Cells are specified if they develop according to their normal fate in an isolated and neutral culture. This is in contrast to determination (c) which describes a tissue that will attain its normal fate even when placed in a non-neutral environment, which can induce the development of other structures. Both of these are two distinct steps in the commitment (e) of cells to their fate. Fate (a) describes the final product of the process of cell differentiation, which is an umbrella term that describes the process by which a less specialised cell becomes a more specialised cell (d). These concepts were most important when classic embryology experiments were the only ones to give us insight into embryology. Since the discovery of morphogens and hox genes and their role in cell differentiation, the importance of these concepts has declined.

Answer 6: EMQ

See *Anatomy at a Glance*, 3rd edn (The arteries of the abdomen).

(1) **E.** The free border of the lesser omentum contains the portal triad: the hepatic artery, common bile duct and the portal vein, and forms the anterior border of the epiploic foramen (of Winslow). If the cystic artery continues bleeding after a cholecystectomy, haemostasis can be achieved by compressing the hepatic artery within the free border of the lesser omentum between two fingers.

(2) **H.** The third part of the duodenum is related anteriorly to the superior mesenteric artery and posteriorly to the aorta. In rare circumstances the duodenum can be compressed between the two vessels, causing obstruction. This is known as the SMA syndrome. Predisposing factors include surgery for scoliosis and drastic weight loss leading to loss of the fat pad at the origin of the SMA that normally keeps the two blood vessels apart.

(3) **I.** The gastroduodenal artery and the common bile duct form the posterior relations of the first part of the duodenum and are at risk of injury if an ulcer in this area perforates.

(4) **F.** The anus is a watershed region that is supplied superiorly by the superior rectal artery arising from the inferior mesenteric artery, and inferiorly by the middle and inferior rectal arteries from the pudendal artery. The different blood supply reflects the different embryonic origin of the two parts of the anus: the superior part of the anus arises from endoderm and is lined by columnar epithelium, like the rest of the digestive tract, whereas the inferior part of the anus arises from ectodermal tissue and thus is lined by stratified squamous epithelium.

(5) **D.** The three thirds of the oesophagus are supplied by three different arteries. The inferior third, relevant to this clinical vignette, is supplied by the oesophageal branch of the left gastric artery. The middle third is supplied by oesophageal branches directly arising from the aorta and the upper third is supplied by the inferior thyroid arteries.

Answer 7: SAQ

See *Anatomy at a Glance*, 3rd edn (The axilla).

The image above is obtained by magnetic resonance imaging (it is a T2-weighted image). It shows pathology in the supraspinatus muscle and tendon. Advantages include high resolution in soft tissue and thus high sensitivity, no contrast needed and no exposure to ionising radiation. Disadvantages include that MRI is expensive/resource-intensive and cannot be done if the patient has a pacemaker, is very obese or claustrophobic.

Answer 8: MCQ

See *Anatomy at a Glance*, 3rd edn (**The nerves of the lower limb II; and The ankle and foot II**).

(b) The problem described here most likely relates to a mechanical rather than neurological problem that is giving rise to flexor hallucis longus dysfunction. The L5 spinal nerve particularly supplies the *extensor* hallucis longus (c), and damage to the deep fibular nerve results in inability to extend toes and variable foot drop (a). Tibial neuropathies on the other hand result in decreased sensation in the sole of the foot, and weakness in ankle and toe plantarflexion, depending on the level of the injury (d). Fractures may cause pain and limited movement, but this will not be direction specific and the patient would be unlikely to bear weight (e).

Answer 9: MCQ

(c) The skin over the back is innervated by a cutaneous branch of the posterior ramus of T3, which is not a named nerve. Both the anterior and posterior ramus arise from the mixed spinal nerve of T3. The anterior ramus gives rise predominantly to the third intercostal nerve which has lateral and terminal cutaneous branches that supply the skin overlying the lateral and anterior chest wall.

Answer 10: SAQ

Figure 1.9 shows a urogram, which is obtained by delivering contrast to the ureters and bladder and taking an X-ray (1). It can be

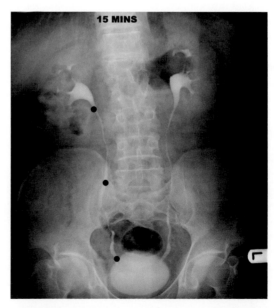

Figure 1.9 Urogram. Black dots denote the places where a kidney stone is most likely to lodge: the ureteropelvic junction, the pelvic brim and the ureteric orifice.

obtained in two ways: in an IV urogram the contrast is administered intravenously, and in a retrograde urogram it is administered using a cystoscope through the urethra (2). The three relatively narrowest regions in a ureter are the ureteropelvic junction (3), the pelvic brim (4) and the ureteric orifice (5). This investigation is no longer routinely performed today as it has been surpassed by spiral CT imaging.

Answer 11: True/False

See *Anatomy at a Glance*, 3rd edn (The mouth, palate and nose).
Waldeyer's ring is formed by mucosa-associated lymphoid tissue (MALT), and forms the initial defence against pathogens entering the respiratory and gastric tracts through the nose and mouth. Its constituents are known as tonsils because, unlike lymph nodes, they are incompletely encapsulated. Waldeyer's ring consists of the nasopharyngeal tonsil (a, 'adenoids'), the paired tubular tonsils (e), the paired palatine tonsils ('the tonsils') and the lingual tonsil (c).

(a) **True**. The 'adenoids' or the nasopharyngeal tonsil is an area of lymphatics found on the posterior surface of the nasopharynx which may increase to obstruct the nasopharyngeal passageway in children, resulting in sleep apnoea.

(b) **False**. The submental lymph nodes can be felt in the anterior triangle of the neck and drain the tongue, lower lip and floor of the mouth. They do not belong to Waldeyer's ring of tonsils.

(c) **True**. Can be found on the posterior aspect of the tongue and are the most inferior of lymph glands forming Waldeyer's ring.

(d) **False**. The submandibular lymph nodes can be felt in the posterior floor of the mouth and are related to the submandibular salivary gland. They drain the upper lip, cheek and parts of the lower lip, gums and tongue.

(e) **True**. The tubular lymphatics surround the pharyngeal entrance to the eustachian tube, and may play a role in recurrent middle ear infections. Due to the blockage of the eustachian tubes, a negative pressure results in the middle ear, triggering a serous effusion that can provide a breeding ground for middle ear infections.

Answer 12: EMQ

See *Anatomy at a Glance*, 3rd edn (Embryology).

(1) **F**. Sensation, including pain sensation, is a function of the dermis, which arises from somatic mesoderm. Somatic mesoderm is formed when the coelom divides the lateral plate mesoderm into two parts. Somatic mesoderm is the dorsal part and forms the body wall lining.

(2) **D**. The combination of craniofacial abnormalities together with cardiac abnormalities is most consistent with a neural crestopathy, which CHARGE syndrome is believed to be. No other embryonic tissue gives rise to such a varied group of tissues.

(3) **H**. The first wave of haematopoiesis occurs in the extraembryonic splanchnic mesoderm of the yolk sac and gives rise to the myeloid linage that includes erythrocytes and neutrophils. However, there appears to be a second intraembryonic source of haematopoietic stem cells, which arises from splanchnic mesoderm, specifically from the aortic, gonad and mesonephros (AGM) region. These cells arise

independently from yolk sac progenitors and both waves of haematopoietic stem cells are needed for the creation of definitive stem cells.

(4) **E**. Neural crest cells are derived from ectoderm – this does not change throughout development. However, initially they are epithelial and epithelial-to-mesenchymal transformation is a key step in the differentiation of neural crest cells. It is important to realise the difference between mesenchyme and mesoderm to answer this question: mesenchyme describes undifferentiated loose connective tissue that is non-epithelial, and does not relate to germ layer origins. Most mesenchyme is mesodermal, but some is ectodermal (neural crest cells).

(5) **G**. Muscles of the axial and appendicular skeleton arise from somitic mesoderm, more specifically from the dermomyotome of somites. It is important not to confuse somitic with somatic mesoderm, which is found in the lateral plate of the embryo.

Answer 13: MCQ

See *Anatomy at a Glance*, 3rd edn (Surface anatomy of the thorax).
(b) This is an echocardiogram of the heart that shows all four chambers. The probe always sits at the meeting point of the two straight edges, which is the top in this case. All four chambers and the two atrioventricular valves can only be visualised from the apex of the heart on the transthoracic echo. The apex in a healthy individual with a normal heart size lies at the fifth intercostal space, midclavicular line.

Answer 14: MCQ

See *Anatomy at a Glance*, 3rd edn (Nerves of the upper limb I and II).
(d) The median nerve supplies most of the muscles in the flexor compartment of the forearm as well as the thenar compartment of the hand, the medial two lumbricals and the skin overlying the thenar compartment. Just below the elbow, the nerve passes between the two bellies of pronator teres, before it gives off the anterior interosseous nerve that supplies the deep muscles of the forearm including flexor pollicis longus and the medial half of flexor digitorum profundus. In pronator teres syndrome, compression of the nerve by pronator teres affects the anterior interosseous nerve and the median nerve below the wrist, as is the case in this patient.

Answer 15: MCQ

See *Anatomy at a Glance*, 3rd edn (The posterior abdominal wall).
(e) The kidneys and adrenal glands lie within a fatty layer within the retroperitoneal space. The kidney is enclosed by a true fibrous capsule (d), which lies in a fatty layer (b) that is contained within the renal fascia (e). The renal fascia is continuous with the transversalis fascia and encloses the suprarenal glands separately and thus creates a plane which allows easy separation of these two organs. Finally the paranephric fat can be found on the outside of the renal fascia (a).

Answer 16: EMQ

See *Anatomy at a Glance*, 3rd edn (The lungs; The thoracic wall II; and The mediastinum I and II).
This is a classic transverse section through the thorax that needs to be recognised. It is at the level of the T3 vertebra, just above the aortic arch, showing the three arteries that supply the upper limbs and the head and neck.

(1) **E.** The thoracic duct inserts into the origin of the left brachiocephalic vein.

(2) **F.** The oesophagus pierces the diaphragm at the level of T10 through an opening in the right crus together with the vagus nerves and the azygos vein.

(3) **A.** The trachea is often described as 'D-shaped' on transverse sections. It acquires this shape from the incomplete cartilaginous rings in its wall, which are open posteriorly.

(4) **C.** The left common carotid artery can be felt as the 'carotid pulse' in the neck. It is derived on both sides from the third branchial arch. The brachiocephalic trunk (D) and both subclavian arteries (B and continuation of D) are derived from the IV branchial arch.

(5) **H.** The spinal cord terminates at the conus terminalis at the level of L1–L2.

Answer 17: True/False

See *Anatomy at a Glance*, **3rd edn** (**The abdominal wall; and Surface anatomy of the abdomen**).

(a) **False.** An indirect inguinal hernia enters the inguinal canal through a patent processus vaginalis which continues through the inguinal canal. By convention, it always arises above the inguinal ligament. If large, it may emerge through the superficial ring, and then it can be felt superior and medial to the pubic tubercle, and may then also enter the scrotum. This is to distinguish it from a femoral hernia, which can be found inferior and lateral to the pubic tubercle.

(b) **False.** The iliohypogastric nerve (L1) does not enter the inguinal canal. It supplies the area superior to the groin. The *ilioinguinal nerve* travels through the inguinal canal where it is susceptible to damage. Unlike all other structures traversing the inguinal ligament, it travels just on the spermatic cord and not within it. It does not descend into the scrotum with the spermatic cord, but separates from the cord at the superficial ring to supply the skin over the anterior scrotum and the root of the penis (or the anterior labia in the female).

(c) **True.** The midinguinal point can be found midway between the pubic *symphysis* and the anterior superior iliac spine. It is the site of the femoral artery. The midinguinal point should not be confused with the midpoint of the inguinal ligament (see d). The needle should be inserted medial to the arterial pulsation. Laterally lies the femoral nerve, which should be avoided. A useful mnemonic is NAVY, the letters stand for nerve, artery, vein and Y-trunks (an *aide-mémoire* for the midline).

(d) **True.** The deep inguinal ring can be found at the midpoint of the inguinal ligament, halfway between the pubic *tubercle* and the anterior superior iliac spine. The inferior epigastric artery passes just medial to the deep inguinal ring. During surgery, it is possible to distinguish indirect hernias, which enter the inguinal canal lateral to the artery through the deep ring, from direct hernias which enter the inguinal canal medially through a defect in Hesselbach's triangle.

(e) **False.** Transversus abdominis arches over the inguinal canal but does not contribute a fascial layer to the spermatic cord, unlike external oblique, which forms the external spermatic fascia, and internal oblique, which forms the cremasteric fascia. The internal spermatic fascia arises from the transversalis fascia.

Answer 18: MCQ

(e) The section shows an osteon, formerly known as a haversian system. It is the hallmark of secondary (lamellar) bone and the building block of cancellous as well as compact bone. It consists of concentrically arranged lamellae that are arranged around a hollow central canal which contains nerve artery and vein.

Answer 19: MCQ

See *Anatomy at a Glance*, **3rd edn (Spinal nerves and cranial nerves I–IV)**.

(c) The gag reflex has an afferent and an efferent limb. The afferents of the posterior tongue and pharynx are carried by the glossopharyngeal nerve, whereas the efferent limb is carried by the vagus nerve. Failure of either the afferent or the efferent limb will result in suppression of the pharyngeal reflex.

Answer 20: SAQ

See *Anatomy at a Glance*, **3rd edn (The hip joint and gluteal region)**.

The acetabulum is the fossa on the lateral aspect of the hip bone that articulates with the femur to form the hip joint, a ball and socket joint (1). The cupped shape of the acetabulum gives the hip joint both stability and weight-carrying capacity, at the same time allowing for a large degree of movement (2). The ilium, ischium and pubis all contribute to the acetabulum (3). The acetabulum is reinforced by the acetabular labrum (4).

The acetabulum is deficient inferiorly, at the acetabular notch (5). From the acetabular notch (and the fossa superior to it) arises the ligamentum teres. Within it passes an artery that supplies the head of the femur in children, but regresses after the fusion of the femoral epiphysis (6).

Answer 21: EMQ

See *Anatomy at a Glance*, **3rd edn (Nerves of the upper limb I and II)**.

(1) **A.** Median nerve injury at the wrist, known as carpal tunnel syndrome, is a common injury and rheumatoid arthritis is an important predisposing factor.

(2) **H.** This is a classic example of 'Saturday night palsy'. The radial nerve supplies the triceps and the wrist and finger extensors. It also supplies the posterior aspects of the forearm and the lateral dorsal aspect of the wrist and the lateral 3½ digits. Sensory loss is variable and complete anaesthesia is rare due to considerable overlap with the other major nerves supplying the upper extremity. Usually only a small area over the first dorsal interosseous muscle between thumb and index finger on the posterior aspect of the hand is affected.

(3) **J.** Paralysis of the ulnar nerve at the elbow is common, as it is exposed behind the medial epicondyle, colloquially known as the 'funny bone'. Ulnar nerve damage at the wrist and elbow predominantly leads to paralysis of most small muscles of the hand other than those supplied by the median nerve. If long standing (not in this case), it results in the characteristic appearance of ulnar nerve injury known as 'claw hand'; the paralysis of the interossei and medial lumbricals leads to an unopposed action of the long digital flexors and extensors, resulting in hyperextension of the metacarpophalangeal joints and flexion of the interphalangeal joints. The difference between ulnar nerve injury at the wrist and elbow is subtle: inability to flex the two medial distal interphalangeal joints

and radial deviation on wrist flexion are seen in lesions at the elbow in addition to those seen at the wrist. A lower trunk brachial plexus injury may also produce a paralysis of the small muscles of the hand, but will not present with the characteristic pattern of ulnar sensory loss.

(4) **D.** Injury of the upper roots of the brachial plexus is also known as Erb–Duchenne paralysis. Muscles supplied by C5 and C6 are paralysed and include supraspinatus, deltoid, biceps and brachialis, resulting in lack of shoulder movement and elbow extension. The forearm is pronated due to paralysis of the biceps, which is the main supinator. This appearance is the classic 'waiter's tip position'.

(5) **C.** The long thoracic nerve supplies serratus anterior, which travels on the surface of the muscle in the midaxillary line where it is prone to injury during knife fights or breast surgery. Its function is to keep the scapula close to the thoracic wall. Together with trapezius, it also rotates the scapula to allow abduction of the shoulder of more than 90°.

Answer 22: MCQ

See *Anatomy at a Glance*, **3rd edn (The mediastinum I)**.
(b) Of the above structures, only the left atrium is a direct relation of the oesophagus. The left ventricle forms the left border of the heart, while the right ventricle is situated anteriorly. The left atrial appendage again lies on the left surface of the heart and is too small to cause significant obstruction. Finally, the thymus is found in the anterior mediastinum. The heart lies between it and the oesophagus.

Answer 23: True/False

See *Anatomy at a Glance*, **3rd edn (Embryology)**.
(1) **True.** Left–right asymmetry is established early in embryology at the primitive node. Extracellular dynein molecules play a role in the establishment of this asymmetry, possibly by the creation of unidirectional flow of a morphogen. Kartagener syndrome involves an abnormality in a gene coding for dynein.
(2) **False.** The syncytiotrophoblast arises from the proliferation of the cytotrophoblast. The decidual reaction is a response by maternal endometrial stroma that is induced by the implanting blastocysts; it results in the accumulation of lipids and glycogen.
(3) **False.** The amniotic cavity arises during the formation of the bilaminar embryonic disc. A little fluid-filled cavity arises between the cells of the inner cell mass, and this develops into the amniotic cavity. Soon thereafter, another fluid-filled layer develops between the extraembryonic mesoderm of the trophoblast, which is the chorionic cavity. Although the chorionic cavity is larger initially, the amniotic cavity soon outgrows it and it is amniotic fluid that is sampled at amniocentesis.
(4) **True.** The human placenta is haemochorial; that is, the chorion/trophoblast directly comes into contact with maternal blood. This is in contrast to the endotheliochorial placenta seen in cats and dogs, where endothelium directly apposes the trophoblastic tissue. In cows, pigs and horses even the maternal endometrial epithelium remains intact, resulting in an epitheliochorial placenta which has three layers separating the maternal and fetal circulation.
(5) **False.** This is almost true, but important exceptions to this rule are the primordial germ cells, which migrate to their final location from the yolk sac.

Answer 24: MCQ

See *Anatomy at a Glance*, **3rd edn (Nerves of the upper limb II)**.
(b) The clinical vignette provides a history of ulnar nerve damage at the level of the wrist: claw hand and weakness of the small muscles of the hand. Sensation on the dorsal 1½ fingers is spared because the dorsal branch of the ulnar nerve arises 5 cm above the wrist and takes a different course. The majority of the ulnar nerve, however, passes medial to the hook of hamate through Guyon's canal, where it is prone to injury during hook of hamate fractures. Hook of hamate fracture is not uncommon in golfers.

Answer 25: MCQ

See *Anatomy at a Glance*, **3rd edn (The pelvis II)**.
(e) The round ligament, which is the lower part of the ovarian gubernaculum, connects the uterus and labia majora and traverses the inguinal canal in the female and may become taut in pregnancy.

The processus vaginalis (c) is an obliterated outpouching of the peritoneum into the inguinal canal, which follows the testes in the male and does not exist in the female. The transverse cervical ligaments (d) are fibromuscular condensations of the pelvic fascia that connect the upper part of the vagina and the cervix to the lateral pelvic walls. The broad ligament (b) is a double layer of peritoneum as it folds over the uterine tubes. It does not connect the uterus with the labia. The suspensory ligament (a) of the ovary is part of the broad ligament. It is a reflection of parietal peritoneum over the ovarian vessels which join the ovaries as they descend from the posterolateral abdominal wall.

Answer 26: EMQ

(1) **C.** Muscles undergo hypertrophy during exercise; that is, they enlarge in size rather than number. A similar process occurs at the zone of hypertrophy at the epiphyseal growth plate.
(2) **B.** The zone of proliferation will contain multiple mitoses amongst chondrocytes, and it is important to remember that this is a normal phenomenon.
(3) **D.** The zone of calcified cartilage is characterised by the absence of chondrocytes but persistence of their calcified matrix in preparation for invasion by osteocytes.
(4) **F.** The dark nuclei signify an area of bone marrow, which will contain areas of white blood cell proliferation and differentiation (basophilic, blue on H&E) and red blood cell synthesis (eosinophilic areas, red on H&E). Erythropoietin is a hormone that stimulates red cell differentiation.
(5) **E.** Osteoblasts invade the osteogenic zone that has been abandoned by chondrocytes. They are found in the osteogenic zone and in mature bone only.

Answer 27: MCQ

See *Anatomy at a Glance*, **3rd edn (The arteries I)**.
(a) The meeting point of the parietal, occipital, frontal and sphenoid bones is also known as the *pterion*. The pterion is a weak point of the skull and is not uncommonly fractured during boxing, golf or bat games. This may damage the *middle meningeal artery*, which runs on the inside of the skull beneath the pterion, resulting in extradural haemorrhage and brain compression. The middle meningeal artery passes through the foramen spinosum together with the less significant meningeal branch of the mandibular division of the trigeminal nerve.

Answer 28: SAQ

See *Anatomy at a Glance*, **3rd edn (The thoracic wall II)**.
The diaphragm originates, at least in part, from the septum transversum (1). After craniocaudal folding, the septum transversum is located adjacent to somites C3–5 (2) and is innervated by them (3). While the septum remains relatively stationary, the dorsal embryo grows, which results in an *apparent* descent of the septum to T8–10 (4), pulling with it the phrenic nerve (5).

Answer 29: MCQ

See *Anatomy at a Glance*, **3rd edn (The nerves of the lower limb I)**.
(c) Hilton's law is the one eponymous law in anatomy that should be known to every doctor as it has great clinical and medico-legal significance. It states that the nerve supply of a joint is the same as the supply of the muscles acting on it. From this, it directly follows that if a muscle crosses two joints (e.g. sartorius crossing both hip and knee joints), one nerve may innervate more than one joint and thus pain may be referred. It is therefore important to always examine the joint below and above the one that is the source of the patient's problems.

Answer 30: True/False

See *Anatomy at a Glance*, **3rd edn (The venous and lymphatic drainage of the upper limb and the breast)**.
Breast cancer is well known for local and distant metastases that can arise years after apparently successful surgery and chemotherapy.

(a) **True**. Metastasis of breast cancer to bone, and especially to thoracic vertebrae, is common due to the direct connection between the intercostal veins draining the breast and the internal vertebral plexus also known as Batson's plexus. In 1940 Batson found that dye injected into the breast of female specimens could be recovered in the vertebral veins.

(b) **False**. Breast cancer may well spread to the liver. However, there is no part of the breast that empties directly into the portal system. Rather, cancer cells travel to the heart and from there to the digestive system to reach the liver.

(c) **True**. Metastasis to the brain via the vertebral plexus is possible anatomically, as the internal vertebral plexus communicates with the occipital sinus superiorly as well as with the intercostal veins that drain the breast. However, arterial metastasis is far more likely and common in the case of breast cancer.

(d) **True**. Metastasis to the opposite breast or opposite axillary lymph nodes is possible due to the overlapping lymphatic drainage of the medial breast.

(e) **False**. Most lymph (80%) from the breast drains into the axilla via the pectoral nodes, though some drainage into the supraclavicular nodes may occur too. Axillary clearance is an effective way of reducing breast cancer recurrence.

2 Anatomy, histology and embryology exam 2

Questions

Question 1: True/False

A 23-year-old man comes to a clinic complaining of double vision. Examination reveals diplopia on looking to the right only. His right eye has limited lateral motion. Which of the following could have caused his examination findings (he may or may not have other cranial nerve involvement)?

(a) Thrombosis of the cavernous sinus
(b) Aneurysm of the internal carotid artery
(c) Tumour pushing on the dorsal brainstem
(d) Fracture of the base of the skull
(e) A sharp object in the superior orbital fissure

Question 2: MCQ

After a successful appendectomy, a surgeon begins suturing the anterior abdominal wall. Superficial to the muscle he encounters a tough membranous layer of tissue. What is the name of this tissue?

(a) Colles' fascia
(b) Scarpa's fascia
(c) Camper's fascia
(d) Deep fascia
(e) Superficial fascia

Question 3: MCQ

A 72-year-old man comes into your clinic complaining of chest pain on the right. He has been feeling unwell for the past 2 days and has developed a temperature of 38.9 °C. For the last day he has been in bed and has been coughing up large amounts of green sputum. The chest pain is worse on inspiration and he points with one finger to the fifth intercostal space on the right in the midclavicular line. You diagnose pneumonia. Inflammation of what part of the pulmonary cavity is responsible for the pain?

(a) Irritation to the visceral pleura by right upper lobe pneumonia
(b) Irritation of the parietal pleura by right middle lobe pneumonia
(c) Irritation of the visceral pleura by right lower lobe pneumonia
(d) Irritation of the right lower lobe bronchus
(e) Irritation of the parietal pleura by right upper lobe pneumonia

Question 4: EMQ

A Bmp
B Fgf4
C Fgf8
D Fgf10
E Hox
F Lrd
G Retinoic acid
H Shh
I Wnt

For each of the scenarios below, choose the most appropriate answer from the list above.

(1) A child is born with polydactyly and three lateral digits which have the appearance of thumbs. A mutation resulting in the overexpression of which molecule will have this effect?
(2) A 20-year-old woman presents with weakness of her right hand with a pain on the medial arm and is found to have a cervical rib. Alteration of the expression of which transcription factor is responsible for the change in the identity of this vertebra?
(3) A 7-year-old child presents with a chest infection and on X-ray imaging is found to have complete situs inversus. Which molecule of the above is the earliest to be involved in the establishment of left–right asymmetry in the mouse model?
(4) Somitic mesoderm differentiates into muscle, bone and dermis. Which of the above molecules, secreted by the dorsal ectoderm and dorsal neural tube, is important for the differentiation of the dermomyotome and thus axial and appendicular muscles?
(5) A transgenic mouse embryo is born without any limbs and with a lung that has failed to form beyond the trachea. Which gene has probably been knocked out?

Question 5: SAQ (5 points)

Describe the anatomy of the anatomical snuffbox and its clinical significance.

Question 6: MCQ

A 23-year-old student injures his knee playing rugby. Figure 2.1 shows an image that is taken for diagnostic purposes. What kind of imaging technique was used to obtain it?

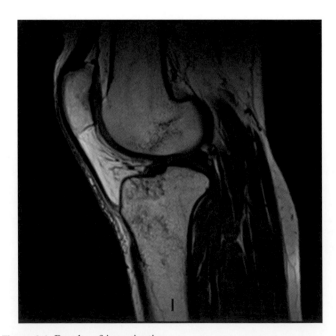

Figure 2.1 Results of investigation.

Medical Sciences at a Glance: Practice Workbook, First Edition. Jakub Scaber, Faisal Rahman and Peter Abrahams. © 2014 John Wiley & Sons, Ltd.

(a) CT
(b) Fluoroscopy
(c) MRI
(d) Ultrasound
(e) Plain radiography

Question 7: SAQ (5 points)

A concerned mother brings her 4-year-old child to the practice and complains that he is still wetting the bed at night. Explain which muscles and nerves play a role in the micturition reflex and how bladder training acts on it.

Question 8: True/False

Which of the following statements regarding Figure 2.2 are true?

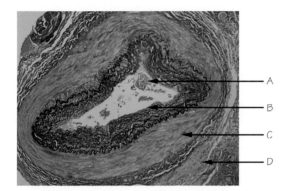

Figure 2.2 Histological section. Reproduced courtesy of Dr Mickhaiel Barrow.

(a) A cardiac surgeon carefully dissects the heart and great vessels during a cardiac transplant operation. The area labelled D is continuous with the epicardium of the heart.
(b) An IV drug user injects cocaine. Its action is on the tissues in area C, which are also under autonomic control.
(c) A biopsy is obtained during the autopsy of a person who died from coronary artery disease. The area labelled B is a stratified squamous epithelium that prevents the formation of thrombi.
(d) The area labelled A contains cells without nuclei.
(e) This section is taken from a large artery close to the heart (such as the aorta).

Question 9: MCQ

A 6-year-old child is admitted to the emergency department with increasing shortness of breath. The child is quietly breathing with considerable effort. He uses accessory muscles during inspiration and expiration, and intercostal and neck muscle movement is easily observed. Which of the following muscles will be assisting forced expiration?
(a) External intercostal muscles, innermost part
(b) External intercostal muscles, outermost part
(c) Internal intercostal muscles, innermost part
(d) Internal intercostal muscles, outermost part
(e) Scalene muscles

Question 10: MCQ

A 47-year-old builder experiences shooting pains in his great toe after lifting heavy loads this morning. Examination reveals altered sensation around the great toe and the anteromedial calf, but no change in muscle tone or power. Which of the following could have led to this presentation?
(a) An infection of the dorsal root ganglion at L5 level by the varicella zoster virus
(b) Compression of the S1 spinal nerve by an intervertebral disc herniation
(c) Compression of the ventral roots of S1 by a spinal cord meningioma
(d) Neuritis (nerve inflammation) of the L5 dorsal ramus
(e) Neuritis (nerve inflammation) of the L5 ventral ramus

Question 11: MCQ

A man undergoes thyroid surgery and is found to have a right recurrent laryngeal nerve which is non-recurrent, due to congenital absence of the structure that it normally winds around. What is the embryonic origin of the structure that the nerve winds around?
(a) First pharyngeal arch
(b) Second pharyngeal arch
(c) Third pharyngeal arch
(d) Fourth pharyngeal arch
(e) Sixth pharyngeal arch

Question 12: EMQ

A Bright-field microscopy
B Transmission electron microscopy
C Scanning electron microscopy
D Phase contrast microscopy
E Fluorescence microscopy
F Positron microscopy
G Polarising microscopy

From the list above, please choose the technique most suited to resolving the problems in the following scenarios.
(1) A scientist looking at the effect of a new chemotherapeutic drug on a cancer cell culture wants to count cell numbers at multiple time points.
(2) A researcher has discovered a new antibody in a mouse model of diabetes. He hypothesises that this antibody may be related or identical to a particular known protein. Which method would be best to demonstrate overlap or correlation between the two?
(3) A 30-year-old patient presents with a tender and erythematous knee. The knee is aspirated and fluid is sent for microscopy. Apart from microscopy and culture for bacteria, the pathologist also wants to exclude the presence of crystals in the aspirate. What technique will be most useful in detecting these organised structures?
(4) A researcher is looking at the effects of an antineoplastic compound and would like to look at the effect of the compound on the structure of microtubules.
(5) A haematologist analyses a bone marrow aspirate that is characterised by an abundance of abnormal lymphocytes. He decides to use immunohistochemical methods to further analyse the sample.

Question 13: True/False

Which of the following statements about urinary tract anatomy are true?

(a) A 55-year-old man presents with swelling of his scrotum, which on examination feels like 'a bag of worms'. He is diagnosed with a varicocele and subsequently also with renal cancer with vascular invasion. This presentation is more likely with a left-sided tumour.

(b) A child is born with a hypoplastic kidney with a reduced number of collecting ducts. The entire human kidney including the collecting ducts is formed from intermediate mesoderm.

(c) During a hysterectomy, a surgeon remembers that the ureter is an important relation of the uterine artery and can be injured during clamping of the artery. When dissecting the uterine artery the ureter will be found superior to it.

(d) A 50-year-old man undergoing chemotherapy for Hodgkin's lymphoma develops anuria and an MRI scan shows retroperitoneal fibrosis. The kidneys and ureters will be affected by this condition because they are secondarily retroperitoneal.

(e) A patient presents with abdominal pain and is found to have signs of urine retention. Urethral catheterisation fails. When inserting a suprapubic catheter, the urologist will need to pierce the peritoneum of the anterior abdominal wall.

Question 14: MCQ

During abdominal surgery, the surgeon nicks the spleen accidentally and proceeds to emergency splenectomy. When operating on the spleen, which structure that lies against the hilum of the spleen must he carefully dissect?

(a) Tail of the pancreas
(b) Second part of the duodenum
(c) Third part of the duodenum
(d) Ureter
(e) Uterus

Question 15: SAQ (5 points)

Describe the development of the thyroid and its relation to neck lumps.

Question 16: EMQ

A Allantois
B Dorsal mesentery
C Umbilical vein
D Umbilical artery
E Yolk sac
F Mesonephric duct
G Metanephric duct
H Paramesonephric duct
I Metanephros
J Cloaca
K Ductus venosus
L Ventral mesentery
M Vitelline duct

For each of the scenarios below, choose the most appropriate answer from the list above.

(1) A 15-day-old infant is brought in by his mother because she noticed that he was leaking urine from his belly button. Which embryonic structure has remained patent?

(2) A 7-year-old child is brought in by her father because she has been complaining of stomach aches. After taking a history and examination, the surgeon decides to do a laparotomy. He finds an inflamed outpouching of the ileum 2 feet from the ileocaecal junction. Which embryological structure is the outpouching derived from?

(3) A 34-year-old woman with Crohn disease is rushed to the emergency CT following a bout of severe abdominal pain 3 h earlier. The CT shows inflammation of the terminal ileum and free air under the right diaphragm. A thin membrane between the liver and the anterior abdominal is clearly visible. What is the embryological origin of that membrane?

(4) A 3-year-old girl comes in with her fifth urinary tract infection in the same year. An ultrasound of the abdomen shows a duplicate ureter with considerable reflux. Duplication of which embryonic structure leads to this presentation?

(5) A young married woman is attending an infertility clinic and her initial ultrasound shows one uterine tube missing and no cornua on that same side of the uterus. Which embryological structure did not develop normally?

Question 17: MCQ

An intestinal biopsy is taken and reported as normal. As part of a research project, the tissue is analysed by transmission electron microscope (Figure 2.3).

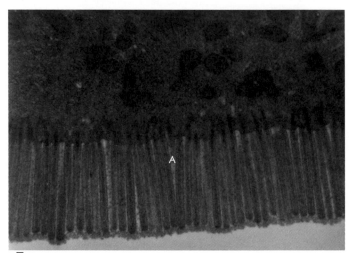

100 nm

Figure 2.3 Electron microscopy image of intestine. Reproduced from Rippel Electronmicroscope Facility at Dartmouth University, Dartmouth College, Hanover, New Hampshire, USA.

What is the name of the structures labelled A?
(a) Microvilli
(b) Villi
(c) Cilia
(d) Flagella
(e) Adhesion proteins

Question 18: MCQ

An elderly lady presents with forearm deformity and she is diagnosed with a fracture of the radius and distal subluxation of the ulna, known as a Galeazzi fracture. The direct articulation of the ulna with which of the following will thus be disrupted?

(a) Lunate
(b) Radius
(c) Scaphoid
(d) Triquetral
(e) All of the above

Question 19: SAQ (5 points)

A 53-year-old woman who has had three children comes to your office complaining that she can feel a lump coming out of her vagina. Examination reveals vaginal prolapse. Which structures normally hold the vagina in place?

Question 20: MCQ

During cardiac transplantation, a surgeon incises the pericardium and separates the aorta and pulmonary artery from the vena cava, by using an existing anatomical division between the two. Which of the following allows effortless separation and clamping of the great vessels?
(a) Foramen ovale
(b) Infundibuloventricular crest
(c) Oblique pericardial sinus
(d) Sternopericardial ligament
(e) Transverse pericardial sinus

Question 21: EMQ

A Vagus nerve
B Phrenic nerve
C Superior laryngeal nerve
D Recurrent laryngeal nerve
E Sympathetic trunk
F Hypoglossal nerve
G Glossopharyngeal nerve
H Ansa cervicalis
I Accessory nerve

For each of the scenarios below, choose the most appropriate answer from the list above.
(1) A 56-year-old builder who smoked for 40 years comes to see his general practitioner because his wife noted that he has a droopy right eyelid. The GP also notes that his right pupil is constricted and finds that the skin on the right side of his face is dry compared with the left. He is sent for an emergency CT. Which nerve has most probably been affected?
(2) During a carotid endarterectomy, a surgeon incises the carotid sheath. As she ties off the carotid artery, which nerve could be damaged during the course of this operation?
(3) After a thyroidectomy, a 35-year-old patient complains of a change in voice. He feels that his singing has got worse and that he keeps missing higher pitched sounds. Which nerve is likely to have been injured?
(4) A 46-year-old patient who has come to see the cardiologist complains of recurrent fainting episodes that have occurred especially whenever she wants to cross the street. The cardiologist connects her to a cardiac monitor, and by massaging her neck finds a marked decrease in her heart rate. Which nerve carries the information from the neck to the brain?

(5) Which nerve supplies the thyrohyoid, which is involved in the depression of the hyoid bone when opening the mouth?

Question 22: True/False

A 52-year-old man with rheumatoid arthritis presents with a flat foot and pain. Which of the statements below about the arches of the foot is true?
(a) The arches of the foot shorten the time that the impact from the floor is transmitted to the pelvis and spine during the stance period.
(b) The deltoid ligament plays a key role in stabilising the medial longitudinal arch.
(c) Dysfunction of the tibialis posterior muscle and tendon results in rigid (irreversible) pes planus.
(d) Dysfunction of the spring ligament results in rigid (irreversible) pes planus.
(e) The spring ligament extends between the talus and calcaneus.

Question 23: MCQ

A 46-year-old man sustained an abdominal gunshot wound a few months earlier which has been operated on and has healed well. However, he now complains of difficulty with ejaculation, while his erections have remained normal. Which of the following nerves was probably injured by the gunshot?
(a) Greater splanchnic nerves
(b) Lesser splanchnic nerves
(c) Least splanchnic nerves
(d) Lumbar splanchnic nerves
(e) Pelvic splanchnic nerves

Question 24: MCQ

A 34-year-old woman presents with her knee joint giving way after she twisted her knee during a hockey game. What is the most important factor in ensuring knee joint stability?
(a) Joint capsule
(b) Intracapsular ligaments
(c) Extracapsular ligaments
(d) Muscles
(e) Bones

Question 25: MCQ

A 36 year old attends the emergency department for an ankle sprain and is found to have highly asymmetrical pupils. The larger pupil does not react to light and accommodation is slowed. Degeneration of fibres in which ganglion could have caused this presentation?
(a) Ciliary
(b) Mandibular
(c) Otic
(d) Pterygopalatine
(e) Superior cervical

Question 26: SAQ (5 points)

A 45-year-old alcoholic presents with recurrent central abdominal pain radiating to the back. A CT of the abdomen is performed. Identify the level of the section in Figure 2.4 and label the numbered arrows.

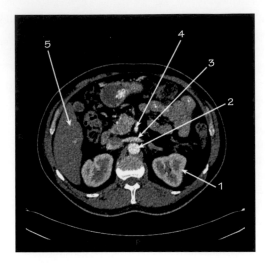

Figure 2.4 CT abdomen.

Question 27: MCQ
An infant is found to have a murmur on initial examination, which on echocardiography turns out to be a defect in the membranous ventricular septum. What is the embryonic origin of the missing septum?
(a) Endoderm
(b) Lateral plate mesoderm
(c) Neural crest cells
(d) Somitic mesoderm
(e) Septum transversum

Question 28: EMQ
A Pseudostratified epithelium
B Simple squamous epithelium
C Simple columnar epithelium
D Simple cuboidal epithelium
E Stratified squamous epithelium
F Stratified cuboidal epithelium
G Stratified columnar epithelium
H Transitional epithelium

For each of the scenarios below, choose the most appropriate answer from the list above.
(1) A 55-year-old man complains of acid reflux and weight loss. He is referred for endoscopy which shows metaplasia of the lower oesophagus. What epithelium can normally be found in the oesophagus?
(2) During a hysterectomy a surgeon is worried about bladder damage. He repairs the potential defect and sends a small amount of damaged tissue for analysis. What type of epithelium would uniquely identify tissue from the urinary tract?
(3) A nasal polyp is sent for histological analysis, as the surgeon is worried about the possibility of a neoplasm. What type of epithelium does the normal nasal mucosa exhibit?
(4) During an endoscopy a biopsy is taken from the duodenum. What epithelial structure will it exhibit?
(5) A woman comes for a cervical (Papanicolaou) smear. The scrapings from the smear come from what kind of epithelium?

Question 29: MCQ
A histological specimen (Figure 2.5) is taken labelled only "gut"

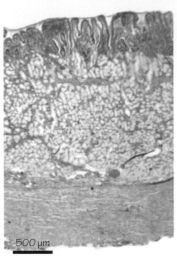

Figure 2.5 Histological specimen of the gut. Reproduced with permission from Peckham M (2011) *Histology at a Glance*. Oxford: Wiley-Blackwell.

What is the likely origin of this specimen?
(a) Oesophagus
(b) Duodenum
(c) Terminal ileum
(d) Colon
(e) Anus

Question 30: True/False
A surgeon performs a laparoscopy for recurrent pelvic pain. Which of the following statements about the relations of the pelvic organs in the peritoneal cavity are true?
(a) Ovaries are covered by peritoneum and are suspended on a mesentery, the suspensory ligament of the ovary.
(b) Fallopian tubes are intraperitoneal.
(c) The fimbrial part of the fallopian tube is also known as the isthmus.
(d) The broad ligament is a mesentery.
(e) Part of the anterior vaginal wall can be visualised with an abdominal laparoscope.

Answers to Exam 2

Answer 1: True/False
See *Anatomy at a Glance*, 3rd edn (Cranial nerves VI–XII).
The inability to abduct the eye laterally suggests paralysis of the lateral rectus, which is supplied by the abducent nerve. The abducent nerve has a long course.
(a) **True.** The abducent nerve is usually the first nerve to be affected by thrombophlebitis, as it is the only nerve passing through the lumen of the cavernous sinus.
(b) **True.** In the lumen of the cavernous sinus the nerve passes in close proximity to the internal carotid artery, by which it can be compressed.
(c) **False.** VI arises from the ventral surface of the junction between the pons and midbrain, and is thus *not* affected by a tumour compressing the dorsal brainstem (initially). The only nerve to exit the brainstem dorsally is the trochlear nerve.
(d) **True.** On emerging from the brainstem, VI passes anteriorly on a long course over the clivus where it can be damaged by fractures of the base of the skull or raised intracranial pressure.
(e) **True.** Together with cranial nerves III, IV and V1, VI traverses the supraorbital fissure where it can be compressed or injured.

Answer 2: MCQ
See *Anatomy at a Glance*, 3rd edn (The abdominal wall).
(b) The membranous layer superficial to external oblique is Scarpa's fascia, which is the membranous part of the superficial fascia of the lower abdominal wall. This membrane is of clinical significance as it is sutured using a continuous suture before suturing the skin, using the toughness of the fascia to bring the wound closer together and achieve a better cosmetic result. Although technically superficial fascia (e) is correct, it refers to both the membranous (b) and fatty (c) components, so (b) is more precise. There is *no deep fascia in the abdomen* or chest because the abdomen and chest need to be flexible to allow for substantial movements during respiration.

Answer 3: MCQ
See *Anatomy at a Glance*, 3rd edn (The pleura and airways; and Surface anatomy of the thorax).
(b) To answer this question, you need to integrate two facts. First, the pain receptors for the chest are located on the parietal side of the pleura, while the visceral pleura (a, c) lining the lungs is sparsely innervated with sensory fibres and generally void of pain receptors. Second, the transverse fissure, which marks the border of the upper and middle lobes on the right, is found anteriorly at the level of the fourth costal cartilage. Our patient experiences pain below that, which must be in the middle lobe (b). The lower lobe has no surface adjacent to the anterior chest wall. Irritation of a bronchus (d) may produce a dull ache in the centre of the chest. This will, however, not localise to a specific point on the chest wall.

Answer 4: EMQ
(1) **H.** Dorsal–ventral patterning of the limb buds is regulated by the zone of patterning activity which secretes sonic hedgehog (Shh) as its main morphogen. Both the concentration and duration of expression of Shh determine the identity of the digits. Overexpression of Shh can result in polydactyly and conversion of more than one digit to thumb identity.
(2) **E.** Establishment of craniocaudal identity of the various vertebrae is established by Fgf and retinoic acid by the action of the somitogenesis clock. These morphogens induce the expression of specific Hox genes at various levels, combinations of which determine vertebral identity at every level. Losses or gains of Hox expression can influence and caudalise or cranialise vertebrae, such as is the case with cervical ribs.
(3) **F.** The gene product of left–right dynein (Lrd) is a dynein that is thought to be responsible for motility of cilia that are found at the primitive node of the mouse embryo. This motility is thought to provide the basis for the establishment of a gradient from right to left that is the initial step in the establishment of left–right asymmetry. Although other genes from the list may be involved in the establishment of left–right asymmetry (e.g. Shh), they are downstream of Lrd. In humans, Kartagener syndrome is a condition characterised by situs inversus and the defective gene also codes for a dynein.
(4) **I.** Wnt molecules, secreted by the ectoderm and dorsal neural tube, play a major role in the establishment of the dermomyotome. The sclerotome, on the other hand, develops under the influence of Shh, which is secreted by the notochord and the ventral neural tube.
(5) **D.** Fgf10 is particularly important in limb outgrowth initiation and Fgf10 knockout mice are amelic. Fgf10 is also an essential chemotactic factor that promotes branching morphogenesis during lung development. Although many genes participate in the establishment and sustaining of limb outgrowth, Fgf4 knockout mice have normal limb growth and Fgf8 mice have reduced limb outgrowth, and neither has a similar effect on lung development.

Answer 5: SAQ
See *Anatomy at a Glance*, 3rd edn (The carpal tunnel and joints of the wrist and hands).
The anatomical snuffbox (Figure 2.6) is demarcated by the extensor pollicis longus on the dorsal side (1) and the tendons of extensor pollicis brevis and adductor pollicis longus on the medial side (2). Its floor is formed by the scaphoid (3), and it is crossed by the

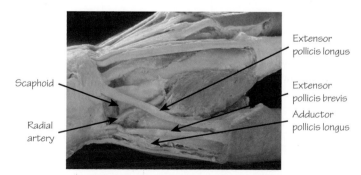

Figure 2.6 The anatomical snuffbox. Reproduced with permission from Abrahams PH, Craven JL and Lumley JSP (2005) *Illustrated Clinical Anatomy*. London: Hodder Arnold.

superficial branch of the radial nerve (4). It contains the radial artery (5).

Clinically the snuffbox is useful in evaluating fractures of the scaphoid, which are characterised by tenderness in the anatomical snuffbox (6).

Answer 6: MCQ

(c) This is an MRI of the knee, which is T1 weighted; both bone and soft tissue have high signal. The high signal of bone may make you confuse the scan with a CT, but this would not have such contrast and signal within soft tissue (a). The image is clearly a sagittal section so neither plain radiography nor fluoroscopy is an option (b, e). Finally, the image does not look like an ultrasound image, which would give an image with few superficial tissues that expand in a triangle towards deep tissue (d).

Answer 7: SAQ

See *Anatomy at a Glance*, 3rd edn (The pelvic viscera).

Continence is achieved by the action of the circular sphincter urethrae muscle, which surrounds most of the urethra in the female and is distal to the prostatic urethra in the male (1), and the sphincter vesicae muscle which is a circular thickening of the detrusor at the bladder neck and can hold the urine long term (2). Both these muscles are usually contracted to keep urine in the bladder. Their relaxation can be effected by the pelvic splanchnic nerves, which are parasympathetic nerves arising from S2, 3 and 4 (3).

The pelvic splanchnic nerves also carry information about bladder distension to the spinal cord. In a child, the signalling of distension of the bladder above 300 mL results in activation of the micturition reflex (4): the afferent signal activates the parasympathetic motor efferents that result in relaxation of the vesical and urethral sphincters and the contraction of the detrusor muscle of the bladder (5).

Toilet training results in wilful suppression of the micturition reflex by neurons originating in the cerebral cortex (6).

Answer 8: True/False

The image depicts the cross-sectional histology of a blood vessel.

(a) **False**. The tunica adventitia, labelled D, is the outermost layer of blood vessels. It contains connective tissue and vasa vasorum, small blood vessels supplying the adventitia and media of the larger blood vessels. It is continuous with the fibrous pericardium of the heart. The epicardium, also known as the visceral pericardium, is only found around the heart and continuous with the parietal pericardium.

(b) **True**. The tunica media contains muscle and connective tissue in varying proportions. Cocaine acts on vascular smooth muscle by inhibiting the reuptake of norepinephrine and thus acts like a sympathomimetic. Except for very few exceptions under parasympathetic control, the majority of vascular smooth muscle is under sympathetic control and will respond to the presence of cocaine.

(c) **False**. B labels the endothelium, not epithelium. Endothelium is always simple squamous.

(d) **True**. Red blood cells do not contain any nuclei.

(e) **False**. Arteries close to the heart contain predominantly elastic tissue in the form of multiple sheets, or lamellae. The tissue predominating in this section is muscle, which is mainly found in distal arteries and arterioles, and helps to control blood flow under the control of the autonomic nervous system.

Answer 9: MCQ

See *Anatomy at a Glance*, 3rd edn (The thoracic wall II).

(d) Only the outermost part of the internal intercostal muscles plays a role in expiration, while all remaining muscles are muscles of inspiration.

Answer 10: MCQ

See *Anatomy at a Glance*, 3rd edn (The spinal cord).

(a) Although this story in a builder is most likely to be due to intervertebral disc herniation, any pathology affecting the nerve supply to the L5 dermatome may result in a similar presentation. Herpes zoster affects the dorsal root ganglion, which contains the cell bodies of *all* somatic sensory fibres from L5, and thus can result in the described distribution of pain which will precede the typical rash. The S1 dermatome encompasses the heel and not the great toe, excluding answers b and c. The L5 dorsal ramus is a mixed nerve arising from the L5 spinal nerve but, like any other dorsal ramus, never contributes to limb nerves and only supplies the back muscles and the skin overlying them (d). Finally, injury to the ventral ramus of L5 (e) (which contributes to the lumbosacral plexus) will result in the described distribution of pain, but since it is a mixed sensory and motor nerve, the patient may also experience motor symptoms.

Answer 11: MCQ

See *Anatomy at a Glance*, 3rd edn (Head and neck, developmental aspects).

(d) On the right, the recurrent laryngeal nerve winds around the right subclavian artery which is a derivative of the fourth aortic arch. If the arch is congenitally absent or regresses, the subclavian artery arises directly from the aorta and the recurrent laryngeal nerve is non-recurrent, which occurs in approximately 1% of the population.

Answer 12: EMQ

(1) **D**. Phase contrast microscopy allows the visualisation of tissue without the need for fixation or staining as it uses a lens system that produces contrast using the differential interference produced by various tissues. It thus allows visualisation of live tissues such as cell cultures.

(2) **E**. Although most immunohistochemistry can be visualised using bright field microscopy, this particular scenario is better addressed using fluorescent microscopy. Modern fluorescent microscopes allow staining with multiple antibodies which are then labelled using compounds that fluoresce at different wavelengths. These images can then be read off at different

wavelengths and added to show any potential overlap or co-localisation of molecules.

(3) **G**. Polarising microscopy is useful for the detection of highly organised tissues and molecules, including collagen, microtubules and crystals. In the case of synovial fluid aspirates, it helps to distinguish gout from pseudogout. Their crystals are positively and negatively birefringent under polarising light, respectively.

(4) **B**. The superstructure of microtubules can only be visualised by transmission electron microscopy, as all other techniques will not have sufficient resolving power.

(5) **A**. Bright field microscopy remains the most important and effective tool available to the pathologist today, and its applications have been greatly expanded by the use of immunohistochemistry. The use of bright field microscopy in this setting is sufficient.

Answer 13: True/False
See *Anatomy at a Glance*, 3rd edn (The posterior abdominal wall; The perineum; and Abdomen, developmental aspects).

(a) **True**. Varicoceles due to renal cell carcinoma are more common on the left due to the anatomical differences in the venous drainage of the gonads between the two sides of the body. The right gonadal vein directly drains into the IVC, whereas the left gonadal vein drains into the left renal vein. Invasion of the left renal vein by renal cell carcinoma may cause obstruction of this tributary, resulting in varicocele.

(b) **True**. Although the kidney forms from two different developmental structures, both the metanephric bud and the metanephric blastema originate from intermediate mesoderm.

(c) **False**. The ureter passes inferior to the gonadal artery and also inferior to the vas in males and the uterine artery in females, (Mnemonic: 'Water flows under the bridge'.)

(d) **False**. The kidneys and ureters are *primarily* retroperitoneal. However, both the kidney and ureters are covered by peritoneum and thus visible from within the abdominal cavity. Retroperitoneal fibrosis is a rare but serious condition that can be idiopathic, but can also follow the administration of chemotherapy or MRI contrast medium.

(e) **False**. When filling, the bladder will lift the peritoneum off the anterior abdominal wall, so that the anterior surface of the bladder is always free of peritoneum. When the bladder is voided, the peritoneum returns to its previous position on the anterior abdominal wall; thus inserting a suprapubic catheter when the bladder is empty inserts it into the abdominal cavity and risks injuring bowel.

Answer 14: MCQ
See *Anatomy at a Glance*, 3rd edn (The pancreas and spleen).

(a) The tail of the pancreas is an important relation of the spleen lying against its hilum. The spleen has the following other relations: the diaphragm posteriorly, stomach anteriorly, left kidney medially and splenic flexure inferiorly. The second and third parts of the duodenum lie to the right of the midline and centrally respectively (b, c), whereas the ureter and the hilum of the kidney are isolated from the spleen as the left kidney lies medially in relation to the spleen (d). The non-gravid uterus is in the pelvis (e).

Answer 15: SAQ
See *Anatomy at a Glance*, 3rd edn (Head and neck, developmental aspects).

The thyroid gland begins its development at the base of the tongue, where its origin is marked by the foramen caecum (1). It then travels inferiorly along the midline along the thyroglossal duct to reach its final destination over the second and third tracheal rings (2). Ectopic thyroid tissue may be present anywhere along its path of migration, and thyroglossal duct cysts should be considered in the differential for midline lumps in the neck (3). Because thyroglossal duct cysts are in communication with the tongue, they can be seen to move if the patient sticks out their tongue (4). Remnants of thyroid tissue can also often be found at the foramen caecum within the posterior tongue, where they are most often asymptomatic (5), but can also descend further than the thyroid isthmus, forming a retrosternal goitre (6).

Answer 16: EMQ
See *Anatomy at a Glance*, 3rd edn (Abdomen, developmental aspects).

(1) **A**. The allantois connects the urogenital sinus with the umbilicus. The lower part of the allantois fuses with the urogenital sinus to form the bladder. The upper part of the allantois obliterates and forms the fibrous urachus, which travels on the anterior abdominal wall in the midline within a peritoneal fold known as the median umbilical fold. Rarely, the urachus may still have a patent lumen at birth, thus leaking urine through the umbilicus, which requires surgical attention.

(2) **M**. The vitelline duct forms the connection between the midgut and the yolk sac. This duct forms the axis for rotation of the midgut and later disappears completely in most individuals. In some, it may persist as a patent duct resulting in an umbilical fistula, or may persist only as an outpouching of the ilium, which is liable to inflammation and also known as Meckel's diverticulum.

(3) **L**. The thin membrane is a double fold of peritoneum that extends from the anterior abdominal wall to the liver and is known as the falciform ligament. It is a remnant of the ventral mesentery which extends from the foregut to the anterior abdominal wall. As the liver develops within the ventral mesentery, the part of the mesentery anterior to the liver becomes the falciform ligament whereas the part connecting the liver and stomach becomes the lesser omentum. The falciform ligament becomes visible on CT scans if the right subphrenic space is filled with fluid or air, as is the case in ascites or after a bowel perforation.

(4) **G**. The proximal urinary tract develops from a bud that originates from the mesonephric duct. This bud is known as the metanephric duct and forms the ureter, pelvis and collecting tubules of the kidney. The metanephric bud grows into the metanephros, which is a cap of mesodermal tissue found in the dorsal wall of the embryo. The metanephros forms the remainder of the kidney.

(5) **H**. The uterus is derived from the fused caudal parts of the paramesonephric ducts, which also form the upper part of the

vagina. The cranial parts of the paramesonephric ducts form the uterine tubes. Failure to develop the paramesonephric duct or its regression during development on one side will result in the clinical picture described.

Answer 17: MCQ

(a) The structures are little projections of cytoplasm (only 1 μm long) visible by electron microscopy – these are microvilli. Villi are much larger structures, consisting of many hundreds of cells whose epithelium is covered by microvilli. Together, microvilli and villi form an increased surface area for absorption of nutrients from the gut. Cilia as well as flagella are much longer than microvilli (up to 10 μm) and visible by light microscopy. They can be found on respiratory epithelium and can be distinguished by the presence of microtubules. In humans, flagella are virtually indistinguishable from cilia, but can be found in sperm, for example. Larger proteins can be visible as dots on transmission electron micrographs.

Answer 18: MCQ

See *Anatomy at a Glance*, 3rd edn (The carpal tunnel and joints of the wrist and hand).

(b) Although there is probably some functional contribution of the ulna to the wrist joint, it is anatomically not a part of the wrist joint. Distally, the ulna directly articulates only with the radius at the distal radioulnar joint which is a pivot synovial joint and includes the triangular fibrocartilaginous disc. The disc articulates with the radius and ulna but distally also with the lunate and triquetral bones. A Galeazzi fracture arises from a high-impact fall on the outstretched hand. Both the fracture and the dislocation at the radioulnar joint need to be addressed surgically.

Answer 19: SAQ

See *Anatomy at a Glance*, 3rd edn (The pelvis I and II).
The upper part of the vagina (as well as the cervix of the uterus) is supported by the transverse cervical, pubocervical and sacrocervical ligaments (1). These ligaments are condensations of fascia on the superior surface of the levator ani muscle which further supports the superior part of the vagina (2). The middle part of the vagina is supported by the urogenital diaphragm (3), whereas the lower part of the vagina is supported by the perineal body (4). The levator ani muscle also inserts into the perineal body, and thus also acts to support the lower part of the vagina (5).

Answer 20: MCQ

See *Anatomy at a Glance*, 3rd edn (The heart I).
(e) The transverse pericardial sinus is a reflection of pericardium that arises due to the degeneration of the mesocardium during cardiac development and creates a communication between the anterior and posterior parts of the pericardial sac in between the superior vena cava posteriorly and the aorta and pulmonary trunk anteriorly. This is used in cardiac transplantation as it allows easy connection of the patient to a bypass machine. The oblique sinus (c) is a blind-ended pocket on the posterior aspect of the heart. The foramen ovale (a) separates the two atria, and the infundibuloventricular crest (b) can be found on the inside of the right

ventricle, separating the ventricle proper from its outflow tract. The sternopericardial ligament (d) attaches the fibrous pericardium to the sternum.

Answer 21: EMQ

See *Anatomy at a Glance*, 3rd edn (Cranial nerves VI–XII; The sympathetic system; and The arteries I).
(1) **E.** The sympathetic trunk provides the only sympathetic supply in the head via the superior cervical ganglion. It dilates the pupil, provides half of the innervation to the levator palpebrae superioris and also supplies sweat glands and arteriolar sphincters in the skin of the head. In this patient the damage to the sympathetic trunk has probably occurred in the root of the neck due to a Pancoast tumour of the apex of the lung, resulting in Horner's syndrome – meiosis, ptosis and anhidrosis.
(2) **A.** The carotid sheath contains the common carotid artery, the internal jugular vein and the vagus nerve.
(3) **C.** During thyroid surgery, both the superior laryngeal nerve and the recurrent laryngeal nerve are prone to injury. They lie in close proximity to the superior and inferior thyroid arteries respectively, and are thus at risk of injury when tying off these arteries. The superior laryngeal nerve supplies the cricothyroid muscle, which is involved in tensing the vocal cords and increasing the pitch of the voice. Thus this patient has most likely suffered an injury to this nerve. The recurrent laryngeal nerve supplies all other muscles of the larynx and injury to it results in a hoarse voice and a motionless vocal cord in the intermediate position.
(4) **G.** The patient is suffering from carotid sinus hypersensitivity. The carotid sinus contains stretch receptors that respond to increases in blood pressure, but are also sensitive to carotid sinus massage. These stretch receptors are innervated by the glossopharyngeal nerve. Stimulation of the carotid sinus results in a brainstem reflex causing slowing of the heart.
(5) **F.** The thyrohyoid is one of the four infrahyoid muscles or strap muscles of the neck. Like the other strap muscles, it is involved in depression of the hyoid bone when opening the mouth and returning the hyoid to its original position after its elevation during swallowing. Unlike the three other strap muscles (omohyoid, sternohyoid and sternothyroid), which are innervated by the ansa cervicalis, the thyrohyoid is supplied by a branch of the hypoglossal nerve. However, this branch is not a true branch of XII, but originates from the C1 ventral ramus that hitchhikes the hypoglossal nerve along most of its course.

Answer 22: True/False

See *Anatomy at a Glance*, 3rd edn (The ankle and foot II).
The arches of the foot (medial and lateral longitudinal and transverse) are very important in locomotion, as they act as shock absorbers and a springboard for the body. Loss of either dynamic or passive support of the arches results in pes planus, or flat foot.
(a) **False.** The arches of the foot *prolong* the impact that arises when the foot rests on the ground. This means that a reduced force is transmitted over a longer time period, protecting the joints above the foot.

(b) **False**. The deltoid ligament is a strong ligament that prevents excessive eversion at the ankle joint which it stabilises efficiently. It does not support the arches of the foot.

(c) **True**. The tibialis posterior tendon is the predominant dynamic support of the transverse plantar arch. After dysfunction or injury to tibialis posterior, the ligaments supporting the transverse arch become the major supports of the transverse arch. Without the dynamic support from its major muscle, the ligaments become lax and the formation of the arches is definitively lost.

(d) **False**. The most important components ensuring the stability of the arches are the muscles. Ligament laxity is often congenital and results in flattening of the foot during weight bearing, but reappearance of the arch on dorsiflexion. The spring ligament mainly supports the medial longitudinal arch.

(e) **False**. The spring ligament stretches between the calcaneus and navicular, but does indirectly support the head of the talus.

Answer 23: MCQ

(d) Ejaculation and erection are controlled by sympathetic and parasympathetic nerves respectively. The parasympathetic innervation to the penis is supplied by pelvic splanchnic nerves (e). The sympathetic nerve supply to the penis arises from the hypogastric plexuses which are supplied mainly by lumbar splanchnic nerves (d). The greater (T5–9, a), lesser (T10–11, b) and least (T12, c) splanchnic nerves are also sympathetic nerves and supply the fore- and midgut.

Answer 24: MCQ

(d) Although all of the above components of the knee joint are essential to provide stability to the joint, the muscles are generally thought to be the most important components in the stabilisation of joints, as their injury or weakness results in damage to the remaining components, which are not able to compensate for the lack of muscle. Degenerative changes in the bone (e) or defects in ligaments (a–c) can often be compensated for by increased muscle mass.

Answer 25: MCQ

See *Anatomy at a Glance*, 3rd edn (Spinal nerves and cranial nerves I–IV).

(a) Anisocoria or asymmetrical pupils are relatively common in the general population. One of the reasons for this is the Holmes–Adie pupil, which is an idiopathic (possibly viral) degeneration of cells in the ciliary ganglion (a). The ciliary ganglion sends parasympathetic fibres to the pupillary muscles that cause pupillary constriction and accommodation. Due to the fact that there are proportionately more nerves that supply accommodation, this action is relatively spared compared with the reaction to light. The superior cervical ganglion (e) supplies sympathetics to the eye and would not result in the above symptoms. The remaining ganglia (b–d) supply parasympathetic fibres to the rest of the head.

Answer 26: SAQ

See *Anatomy at a Glance*, 3rd edn (The posterior abdominal wall). The presence of the renal vein indicates the level of L1–L2 (L2 vertebra is seen). The structures to be identified on the scan are:

(1) Kidney
(2) Aorta
(3) Left renal vein
(4) Superior mesenteric artery
(5) Liver

Answer 27: MCQ

See *Anatomy at a Glance*, 3rd edn (Thorax: developmental aspects).

(c) Whereas the majority of the heart is derived from lateral plate mesoderm in the cranial region of the trilaminar embryo, the membranous parts of the endocardial cushions are derived from neural crest cells, which migrate considerable distances, making this process more prone to failure than the remainder of cardiac development.

Answer 28: EMQ

(1) **E.** The oesophagus has few secretory and digestive functions and is lined by stratified squamous epithelium that protects the oesophagus from abrasion by sharp or hot foods. In gastro-oesophageal reflux disease, the acid reflux can cause a metaplasia of the lower oesophageal epithelium, transforming it into simple columnar epithelium that is also found in the stomach.

(2) **H.** The bladder contains a unique type of stratified epithelium, whose architecture allows considerable stretch. In the resting state the epithelium has five or more layers, whereas when stretched it appears to have only two.

(3) **A.** Upper respiratory epithelium including nasal and tracheal epithelium is pseudostratified; it is a simple columnar epithelium, where every cell adheres to the basement membrane, but which appears stratified.

(4) **C.** The epithelium of the majority of the gastrointestinal tract from the stomach to the upper anus is simple columnar.

(5) **E.** The outer cervix and vagina, in contrast to the uterus, are lined with a stratified squamous epithelium. The cervical smear collects squamous cells from the outer cervix.

Answer 29: MCQ

(b) The specimen shows large villi with branching ducts underneath. The villous structure with glands suggests a secretory function of the epithelium. The particular compound branched tubular structure is only seen in the duodenum. It is easily seen on the image and is also known as Brunner's glands.

Answer 30: True/False

See *Anatomy at a Glance*, 3rd edn (The peritoneum).

(a) **False**. Although often described as intraperitoneal, a more precise term is interperitoneal, as it is the only organ that is found inside the peritoneal cavity without a covering of peritoneum (although parts of the ovary arise from peritoneum). It is merely suspended by a termination of the broad ligament which provides it with blood and nerve supply.

(b) **True**. Fallopian tubes are entirely intraperitoneal in their course and are easily accessible from the abdominal cavity, for example during the resection of an ectopic pregnancy.

(c) **False**. The isthmus is the narrow part of the fallopian tubes that links to the uterus. The infundibulum is the part that opens into the abdominal cavity and is associated with the fimbriae.

(d) **True**. The broad ligament serves as a mesentery for the fallopian tubes and the uterus and is also the origin of the suspensory ligament of the ovary.

(e) **False**. The uppermost part of the *posterior* vaginal wall, known as the fornix, forms part of the wall of the pouch of Douglas. Anteriorly, the peritoneum does not reach the fornix, as the peritoneum directly reflects from the bladder onto the neck of the uterus.

Biochemistry and genetics exam 1

Questions

Question 1: MCQ
While creating a permanent on a student, a hairdresser accidentally spills some ammonium thioglycolate (also known as perm salt) onto the student's skin. The student notices irritation of the skin on that spot a few hours later. Ammonium thioglycolate reduces disulphide bonds, which are formed by which amino acid?
(a) Methionine
(b) Threonine
(c) Tyrosine
(d) Cysteine
(e) Serine

Question 2: MCQ
A dermatologist advises a fair-haired woman to avoid sun exposure and to use barrier cream. What kind of mutations will these steps prevent?
(a) Spontaneous deamination
(b) Pyrimidine dimers
(c) Interferes with DNA polymerase proofreading
(d) Double-stranded breaks
(e) Single-stranded breaks

Question 3: True/False
A 34-year-old depressed patient impulsively takes an overdose of aspirin tablets and presents to hospital. Aspirin has a pKa of 3.8. Assuming it is easily absorbed, which of the following are true?
(a) The substance will work as a buffer in the blood.
(b) The protonated form of the substance will be predominant.
(c) The substance is a weak acid.
(d) The pH of the blood will fall.
(e) The net charge of the acid and conjugate base at physiological pH will be positive.

Question 4: SAQ (5 points)
Describe the phenomenon of genetic imprinting using Prader–Willi and Angelman syndromes as examples.

Question 5: MCQ
When setting up a polymerase chain reaction, the laboratory technician adds the necessary deoxyribonucleotide triphosphates to the reaction mixture. He includes 5 mmol of dCTP and dATP and 10 mmol of dGTP and dTTP. The sequence that will be amplified is known to contain 30% of guanine bases in the code. Which deoxyribonucleotide triphosphate will run out first?
(a) dCTP
(b) dATP
(c) dGTP
(d) dTTP
(e) dCTP and dATP at the same time

Question 6: EMQ
A cyclin A
B cyclin B
C cyclin D
D APC/C
E Retinoblastoma
F E2F
G PTEN
H c-Myc
I p53
J ras
K PKB
L APC

For each question below, choose the correct option from the list above.
(1) A biopsy of a pancreatic cancer is analysed biochemically. It is found that the MAP kinase pathway is inherently activated independent of tyrosine kinase activity. A mutation of which proto-oncogene is responsible?
(2) A researcher is investigating the usefulness of tumour markers for treatment. He notes an elevated PIP_2 and PIP_3, and finds that they have negative predictive value for treatment success. He finds that the elevated PIP levels are caused by the absence of a PIP phosphatase. Which tumour suppressor gene is most probably silenced?
(3) A regular user of a solarium has a skin biopsy, showing an increased level of a tumour suppressor gene. Which tumour suppressor gene is activated by UV light, and can arrest the cell cycle, but can also induce apoptosis by transcriptional activation of *bax*?
(4) A young man with a history of colon cancer in his family arrives for genetic testing. He is predisposed to colon cancer and other cancers because of a mutation in the gene coding for a tumour suppressor protein that normally prevents the translocation of β-catenin to the nucleus. What is the name of that gene?
(5) A 60-year-old man with chronic hepatitis B infection is found to have hepatocellular carcinoma. Multinucleated tumour cells are seen. Hepatitis B virus induces a protein that promotes separation of sister chromatids and exit from M phase. Which protein is inappropriately activated by the virus, and is normally inhibited by the spindle checkpoint?

Question 7: MCQ
A woman with known α-galactosidase A deficiency, a multisystem disorder affecting the kidneys, heart and skin, attends a genetics clinic appointment with her son who is beginning to suffer from the condition. The woman confirms a family history of the disease and remarks that the disease affects men more severely than women. A family tree is drawn up (Figure 3.1). What is the likely pattern of inheritance of this condition?

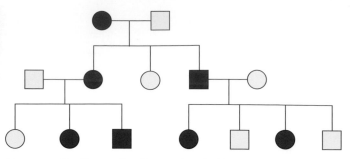

Figure 3.1 Family tree. Family members in blue are affected, those in yellow are unaffected.

(a) Autosomal dominant
(b) Autosomal recessive
(c) Mitochondrial
(d) X-linked dominant
(e) X-linked recessive

Question 8: True/False

A marathon runner has an energy drink. After entering his muscle cells, it is metabolised by hexokinase. Which of the following statements about hexokinase are true?
(a) Hexokinase is inhibited by its product.
(b) Hexokinase has a high K_m but low V_{max}.
(c) Hexokinase catalyses the rate-limiting step of glycolysis.
(d) Hexokinase commits the glucose molecule to the cell.
(e) The reaction catalysed by hexokinase generates ATP.

Question 9: SAQ (5 points)

You are performing a pregnancy test and are using ELISA to detect β-hCG. You have sufficient quantities of anti-β-hCG monoclonal and anti-β-hCG polyclonal antibody for the test. Use diagrams to illustrate how you would perform the test, indicating which antibody type you would use.

Question 10: EMQ

A Ubiquitin
B Pepsin
C Trypsin
D Gastrin
E Bilirubin
F Signal recognition peptide
G C-peptide
H Cholecystokinin
I Alanine aminotransferase
J Glutamate dehydrogenase
K Glutamine synthetase
L Carbamoyl phosphate synthetase I

For each question below, choose the correct option from the list above.
(1) A 45-year-old man comes to the hospital after a binge on alcohol. His liver damage is monitored by the presence of an enzyme, which requires vitamin B_6 as a co-factor. Which enzyme matches this description?
(2) A 44-year-old woman with chronic pancreatitis takes Creon (pancreatin) to replace pancreatic enzymes. Which of the above is part of Creon?

(3) A 67-year-old man takes regular proton pump inhibitors that increase the pH of the gastric contents. The raised pH will inhibit the action of which enzyme?
(4) A 78-year-old man suffering from an atypical dementia characterised by increased gambling and personality changes dies. The autopsy shows inclusions that stain positively for a polypeptide that marks proteins for degradation. What is the name of that polypeptide?
(5) A 23-year-old worker on a hunger strike is rapidly using muscle mass, as his body protein is being recruited as an energy fuel. Which enzyme is responsible for deamination to free the ketone backbone of the degraded proteins?

Question 11: MCQ

A marathon runner is preparing her glucose-based energy drink for the next competition. What other substance should she add to the drink to aid the absorption of the large amount of glucose?
(a) Alanine
(b) Sodium
(c) Caffeine
(d) Chloride
(e) ATP

Question 12: MCQ

A researcher finds different isoforms of glutaminase that seem to be tissue specific. What is the likely explanation of tissue specificity?
(a) Over time mutations accumulate in different tissues, giving rise to different isoforms.
(b) Various tissue types create different proteins by means of alternative splicing.
(c) The enzyme is located at the end of telomeres and is truncated in ageing cells.
(d) An operon is responsible for differential transcription.
(e) Paternal and maternal DNA is different.

Question 13: MCQ

A laboratory technician is measuring substrate levels in a bag of stored fresh red blood cells. Which of the following substrates of glycolysis is uniquely found in red blood cells in high concentrations?
(a) Glyceraldehyde 3 phosphate
(b) 1,3 bisphosphoglycerate
(c) 2,3 bisphosphoglycerate
(d) 2-phosphoglycerate
(e) 3-phosphoglycerate

Question 14: True/False

A 14-year-old girl presents to the emergency department with severe dehydration and reduced consciousness. She is found to have a high blood glucose level and severe ketoacidosis. Which *one* statement about ketones is true?
(a) Ketones are produced mainly by the liver in response to a high NADH level in hepatic mitochondria.
(b) Ketones are transported in the blood via lipoproteins and albumin.
(c) Significant amounts of ketones are derived from β-oxidation of fatty acids in muscle, brain and liver cells.
(d) Production of ketones occurs in the cytosol.
(e) Giving insulin will be therapeutic in this case and will reverse both abnormalities.

Question 15: MCQ

A young infant is noted to be increasingly hypotonic after birth and after 2 weeks develops seizures. The serum ammonia level is raised, suggesting a defect in the pathway that metabolises ammonia. What enzyme catalyses its rate-limiting step?
(a) Argininosuccinate synthase
(b) Argininosuccinate lyase
(c) Carbamoyl phosphate synthetase
(d) Glutamate dehydrogenase
(e) Arginase

Question 16: EMQ

A Vitamin A
B Vitamin B_1
C Vitamin B_2
D Vitamin B_3
E Vitamin B_6
F Vitamin B_{12}
G Vitamin C
H Vitamin D
I Vitamin E
J Biotin

Which vitamin is deficient in the following scenarios?
(1) A 43-year-old alcoholic who also suffered from memory loss is found to have decreased amounts of myelin around the axons with abnormal odd chain fatty acid breakdown.
(2) A malnourished child presents with bruising and bleeding gums. The illness is characterised by abnormal collagen and absence of proline hydroxylation.
(3) A young man on tuberculosis treatment develops a peripheral neuropathy. A co-factor needed for transamination is deficient.
(4) A 48-year-old alcoholic presents with heart failure. Pyruvate levels are elevated in the blood and further increase after administration of glucose. Red cell transketolase function is impaired.
(5) A malnourished 77-year-old alcoholic presents with loose stools, a photosensitive widespread rash and progressive confusion. Levels of NAD breakdown products in the urine are low.

Question 17: MCQ

A 60-year-old woman with symptoms of involuntary movements and increasing mental retardation is diagnosed with Huntington's disease. Her parents are still alive and well, but her family remembers that the patient's maternal grandmother had a similar condition. The patient's mother, who is 89 years old, undergoes genetic testing and is found to be positive for the mutation but has no clinical signs of the disease. This is an example of which of the following?
(a) X-linked inheritance
(b) Autosomal recessive inheritance
(c) Variable penetrance
(d) Anticipation
(e) High recurrent mutation rate

Question 18: SAQ (5 points)

Coupled reactions are common in human metabolism. Give an example of a coupled reaction and explain the advantages of coupled reactions.

Question 19: MCQ

A doctor takes a sample of cerebrospinal fluid (CSF) from a patient with encephalitis. The CSF is sent for amplification via polymerase chain reaction (PCR). Assuming there are 20 viral particles in the aliquot, and that at least 20,000 PCR fragments are needed to read the result, how many cycles of PCR will need to be completed?
(a) 9
(b) 10
(c) 99
(d) 100
(e) 101

Question 20: EMQ

A Fragile X syndrome
B Huntington disease
C Down syndrome
D Edwards syndrome
E Phenotypically normal individual
F Friedreich ataxia
G Kennedy disease
H Turner syndrome
I Patau syndrome
J Klinefelter syndrome

Which conditions are described in these scenarios?
(1) A pathologist looking at a cervical smear finds that there are two Barr bodies in the nuclei.
(2) A child is brought in to the development clinic with weakness and developmental delay. Genetic analysis reveals a gene that has been silenced by a triplet expansion. The condition is autosomal recessive.
(3) A young woman attends fertility clinic with her boyfriend. She has no menstrual periods and upon closer inspection she has an unusually wide chest and a low hairline. She reports frequent ear infections in childhood and karyotyping is abnormal.
(4) An infant is born with a severe ventricular septal defect, clenched hand, club foot and webbing of fingers and toes. Karyotyping shows an additional chromosome 18.
(5) A 45-year-old man attends a neurology clinic with increasing difficulty with eating and swallowing and weakness of his upper limbs. He is found to have muscle wasting and fasciculations. His maternal uncle had a similar illness. Genetic studies show a CAG trinucleotide repeat disorder with toxic gain of function.

Question 21: SAQ (5 points)

A 1 mL suspension of mitochondria is set up to investigate the impact of a new drug on the respiratory chain (Figure 3.2). P_i and succinate are added initially at sufficient quantities. 300 nmol of ADP is added at time point 1. An uncoupler is added at time point 2. The same experiment is repeated but with the addition of the new drug X at the beginning of the experiment.

Calculate the ATP:O ratio for succinate in the control experiment and explain what you can deduce about the action of drug X.

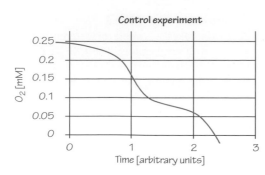
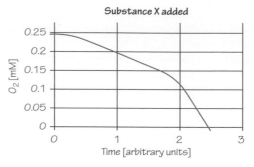

Figure 3.2 Graphs showing the oxygen released over time, before and after the addition of substance X.

Question 22: MCQ

During a prolonged stay in hospital, a 67-year-old woman notices she has become considerably weaker. Her thighs and calves are thinner due to disuse atrophy. Her urine has an increased level of ammonium ions. In what form is ammonia transported from the muscle so it can be directly excreted by the kidneys?

(a) Alanine
(b) Free ammonium ions
(c) Glutamine
(d) Glutamate
(e) Urea

Question 23: True/False

A researcher is trying to find a new selective antibacterial agent. Which of the following mechanisms will be efficacious at interfering with bacterial metabolism?

(a) A compound that inhibits 40S ribosomal subunits
(b) A compound that prevents recognition of the Shine–Dalgarno sequence
(c) A compound that tightly binds ρ factor and prevents its function
(d) An inhibitor of reverse transcriptase
(e) A nucleoside analogue

Question 24: MCQ

A 34-year-old diabetic worried about his health comes for a check-up. His HDL cholesterol levels are high. Which *one* of the following statements is true?

(a) High-density lipoprotein serves as a reservoir of Apo B 100 and Apo E for other lipoproteins.
(b) High-density lipoprotein can esterify cholesterol.
(c) The main function of HDL is to deliver cholesterol to peripheral tissues.
(d) High-density lipoprotein delivers cholesterol to the kidney for excretion.
(e) High-density lipoprotein levels rise with diets consisting of fast food.

Question 25: MCQ

A newborn genetic male (X,Y) is born with female-like genitalia. Cortisol, oestrogen and testosterone levels are low. The infant develops hypertension over the course of months. Which enzyme of steroid hormone synthesis is probably deficient?

(a) 3β-hydroxysteroid dehydrogenase
(b) 17α-hydroxylase
(c) 21α-hydroxylase
(d) 11β-hydroxylase
(e) 5α-reductase

Question 26: SAQ (5 points)

Why is it not possible to replenish glucose stores from fatty acids?

Question 27: MCQ

A mountaineer spends a few months at Mount Everest base camp. His blood tests on return show an increased level of 2,3-bisphosphoglycerate (2,3-BPG). How will his oxygen saturation curve be affected (Figure 3.3)?

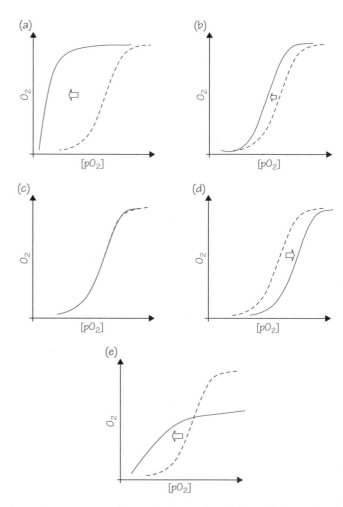

Figure 3.3 Various oxygen saturation curves. The dashed line is the control curve and the solid line was taken after returning from Mount Everest base camp.

Question 28: True/False

A 67-year-old patient begins eating after 3 days of being nil by mouth following a bowel operation. Her glycogen stores are depleted. Which of the following statements are true?

(a) During fasting, glycogen synthase will be predominantly in its phosphorylated form.

(b) Primers are required to commence glycogen synthesis.

(c) Glycogen synthase uses glucose-6-phosphate as a substrate for glycogenesis.

(d) Insulin is an allosteric activator of glycogen synthase.

(e) Glycogen synthase forms $\alpha(1 \rightarrow 6)$ bonds between the non-reducing end of a polysaccharide and activated glucose.

Question 29: MCQ

A 18-year-old girl is diagnosed with systemic lupus erythematosus and decides to enrol in a research study. She is found to have antibodies to snRNPs. This will interfere with which process?

(a) DNA synthesis

(b) Post-transcriptional modification

(c) Post-translational modification

(d) Transcription

(e) Translation

Question 30: EMQ

A Alanine
B Asparagine
C Cysteine
D Glutamate
E Glutamine
F Glycine
G Leucine
H Methionine
I Ornithine
J Proline
K Threonine

For each question below, choose the correct option from the list above.

(1) Within 24 h of fasting, protein catabolism takes place in muscle cells. The product of this catabolism can then be used for gluconeogenesis. Which amino acid forms the link between muscle catabolism and carbohydrate metabolism?

(2) A 64-year-old man with emphysema has a respiratory acidosis with metabolic compensation. The metabolic compensation is achieved by excretion of ammonia into the urine in exchange for bicarbonate reabsorption. What amino acid provides the source for this ammonia?

(3) A laboratory is sequencing a misfolded polypeptide from a cytoplasmic inclusion in a neurodegenerative disease. Which amino acid are they least likely to find in the sequence?

(4) A child with a mutation of one of the urea cycle proteins presents with failure to thrive. She is found to have carbamoyl phosphate synthetase deficiency. The serum concentration of which amino acid will be elevated as a result?

(5) A 30-year-old woman attends the emergency department with flank pain. She is found to have multiple kidney stones composed predominantly of cystine. Which other amino acid will be found in increased quantities in her urine?

Answers to Exam 1

Answer 1: MCQ

See *Medical Biochemistry at a Glance*, 3rd edn (Amino acids and the primary structure of proteins) and *Medical Sciences at a Glance* (Proteins).

(d) Cysteine is the only amino acid that is capable of forming disulphide bonds because it has a thiol (R-SH) group that can form disulphide (S-S) bonds. The only other sulphur-containing amino acid is methionine (R$\sim$S$-$CH$_3$); however, it is not available to form disulphide bonds as it is linked to a terminal methyl residue.

Answer 2: MCQ

See *Medical Biochemistry at a Glance*, 3rd edn (DNA damage and repair).

(b) Ultraviolet light induces pyrimidine dimers. Spontaneous deamination occurs without triggers (a), double-stranded breaks can be caused by ionising radiation (d), while single-stranded breaks are seen with increased temperatures (e).

Answer 3: True/False

See *Medical Biochemistry at a Glance*, 3rd edn (Understanding pH) and *Medical Sciences at a Glance* (Acid–base physiology).

(a) **False**. Buffers have a pK$_a$ that is close to the physiological pH of 7.

(b) **False**. The substance is an acid, and will thus be releasing protons in the blood.

(c) **True**. Although there are no definite rules, it is considered that acids with a pK$_a$ greater than 2 or 3 do not fully dissociate in water and are thus 'weak'. Most acids are weak acids.

(d) **True**. Addition of a substance with a lower pK$_a$ than the physiological pH to blood will result in a lowering of the blood pH.

(e) **False**. The net charge will be negative. Remember that: $pK_a = pH - \log[\frac{A^-}{AH}]$ which can be rearranged as $\frac{[A^-]}{[AH]} = 10^{(pH - pK_a)}$. In our case this means that $\frac{[A^-]}{[AH]} \approx 1500$ at physiological pH; thus an abundance of the conjugate base will result in a net negative charge.

Answer 4: SAQ

See *Medical Genetics at a Glance*, 3rd edn (Genomic imprinting and Dynamic mutation).

Genetic imprinting is a phenomenon by which genes in a child are expressed depending on which parent they have come from (1). This is achieved by silencing of either the maternal or paternal allele, e.g. through methylation (2). Both Angelmsan and Prader–Willi syndromes can arise from deletion of the same area of chromosome 15 (3). The maternal and paternal copies of this area have very different gene expression as a result of imprinting, thus deletion of the area from either chromosome cannot be compensated for by the other (4). In Angelman syndrome the maternal UBE3A gene is deleted, whereas the same gene on the paternal chromosome is silenced by methylation and as a result the gene is not expressed at all (5). In the case of Prader–Willi syndrome it is the paternal gene SNRPN and related genes that are deleted whereas these maternal genes are silenced (6).

Answer 5: MCQ

See *Medical Biochemistry at a Glance*, 3rd edn (Structure of DNA) and *Medical Sciences at a Glance* (DNA and RNA).

(a) Because base pairs are complementary, we know that the strand contains 30% of both guanine and cytosine and 20% of both adenine and thymine. Of the bases included at the lower concentration, cytosine is needed more and will run out first.

Answer 6: EMQ

See *Medical Biochemistry at a Glance*, 3rd edn (The cell cycle) and *Medical Sciences at a Glance* (Cancer biology).

(1) **J**. The MAP kinase pathway is an important pathway activated by growth factors that leads to the transcription of pro-proliferative genes. Ras is a G-protein downstream of the growth factor receptor. Ras is active in its GTP-bound confirmation, but possesses intrinsic GTPase activity which is facilitated by another protein (Ras-GAP). Mutations can result in constitutive activation of Ras (e.g. through loss of GTPase activity), resulting in overactivity of the MAPK pathway.

(2) **G**. PTEN is a PIP$_3$ phosphatase that is involved in the termination of the AKT/PKB pathway. The pathway can be activated by signals such as insulin-like growth factor, causing an increase in PIP$_3$ synthesis. PIP$_3$ activates AKT and PKB which result in the activation of proliferative, synthetic and antiapoptotic pathways. PTEN is a tumour suppressor gene, since its absence facilitates cancer.

(3) **I**. Ultraviolet radiation results in the formation of pyrimidine dimers and is known to cause DNA mutations. The increasing mutations are recognised by dividing cells, and prevent them from passing the cell cycle check points. Proteins such as p53 become active when DNA is damaged and arrest the cell cycle until the damage is repaired.

(4) **L**. The history of colon cancer and the description of the protein's action point to adenomatous polyposis coli (APC), a protein that acts together with GSK3β to phosphorylate β-catenin and thereby mark it for degradation. In the absence of APC function, β-catenin accumulates, translocates to the nucleus and acts as a transcription factor for a variety of genes that have the potential to change the proliferative state of the cell, including c-Myc and cyclin D.

(5) **D**. Anaphase promoting complex (APC/C) is under tight regulation by the spindle check point. Only when all kinetochores are connected to the opposite poles of the mitotic spindle is APC/C activated. A number of viruses over-ride this checkpoint by activating APC/C independently; this includes hepatitis B and orf.

Answer 7: MCQ

See *Medical Genetics at a Glance*, 3rd edn (X-linked and Y-linked inheritance) and *Medical Sciences at a Glance* (Medical genetics).

(d) The condition is clearly dominant, as it is passed down two generations. Note that men can only transmit the disease to every daughter but never to a son. The condition occurs twice as frequently in females as in males. α-Galactosidase deficiency is indeed one of the few rare examples of X-linked dominant diseases. The differential here is autosomal dominant transmission, but the worse phenotype in men points more towards X-linked dominant disease. Given that males can pass on the disease, this makes mitochondrial transmission impossible.

Answer 8: True/False

See *Medical Biochemistry at a Glance*, 3rd edn (**Anaerobic oxidation of glucose by glycolysis**) and *Medical Sciences at a Glance* (**Glucose as a fuel**).

(a) **True**. Glucose-6-phosphate inhibits hexokinase (but not glucokinase in the liver).

(b) **False**. Hexokinase, compared with glucokinase, has a very high affinity for glucose (low K_m) but also a low capacity (low V_{max}).

(c) **False**. Hexokinase catalyses the phosphorylation of glucose to glucose-6-phosphate. This can then undergo multiple fates: glycolysis, glycogenesis or continue in the pentose phosphate pathway.

(d) **True**. Hexokinase 'traps' the phosphorylated glucose molecule as the reaction is essentially irreversible under physiological conditions and the phosphorylated glucose is charged so cannot diffuse out of the cell.

(e) **False**. The initial step in glycolysis *requires* ATP.

Answer 9: SAQ

Enzyme-linked immunosorbent assay (ELISA) is now a key method used in a wide range of tests ordered by doctors. Understanding its principles is important (Figure 3.4).

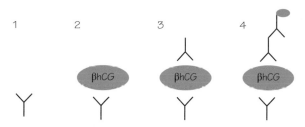

Figure 3.4 Stages involved in enzyme-linked immunosorbent assay (ELISA) testing.

(1) Coat wells with first anti-β-hCG antibody.

(2) Add serum then wash out. Only β-hCG will adhere to the wells.

(3) Add second anti-β-hCG antibody then wash out.

(4) Add anti-F_c antibody which is conjugated to enzyme or pigment to give an indication of β-hCG concentration.

(5) It is better to use the monoclonal antibody for the first stage (see figure 3.4), as this will limit the amount of non-specific binding, and then use the polyclonal for the third stage, to give optimal pick-up and prevent epitope blocking. However, you can also argue that using a polyclonal first will give you maximal pick-up. Using a monoclonal antibody for the third stage will result in a more accurate estimate of the concentration.

Answer 10: EMQ

See *Medical Biochemistry at a Glance*, 3rd edn (**Water-soluble vitamins II**) and *Medical Sciences at a Glance* (**Amino acid metabolism, Upper GI physiology, Amino acid metabolism and Proteins**).

(1) **I**. Transamination reactions catalysed by both ALT and AST reactions require vitamin B_6, as the transfer of the amino group proceeds via this vitamin.

(2) **C**. Creon contains trypsin, which is a serine protease. It also contains lipase (for lipid digestion) and amylase (for starch digestion) and thus mimics pancreatic secretions.

(3) **B**. Pepsin is secreted by gastric chief cells. It is activated by a low pH.

(4) **A**. Ubiquitin is a small polypeptide chain that marks proteins for degradation. In degenerative processes cytosolic accumulation of ubiquitinated proteins may occur when the cell is no longer able to cope with the amount of proteins marked for degradation.

(5) **J**. During protein catabolism, most amino acids are converted to glutamate via transamination. Glutamate is the only amino acid that undergoes rapid oxidative deamination, catalysed by glutamate dehydrogenase. The resulting carboxylic acid is α-ketogluterate, which is a substrate for gluconeogenesis.

Answer 11: MCQ

See *Medical Biochemistry at a Glance*, 3rd edn (**Regulation of glycolysis and Krebs cycle**) and *Medical Sciences at a Glance* (**Lower GI physiology**).

(b) The absorption of glucose by intestinal mucosal cells occurs in the duodenum and ileum, predominantly by way of the sodium-dependent glucose co-transporter 1 (SGLT1).

Alanine is absorbed by a glucose-independent transporter that is selective for neutral amino acids. Like the glucose transporter, it is a sodium-dependent co-porter.

Caffeine is a hydrophobic molecule that traverses the intestinal membrane passively without the help of a transporter down a steep concentration gradient. Its absorption in the gut is almost complete (99%).

Chloride is usually absorbed across the intestinal membrane together with sodium, or follows sodium absorption through an electrochemical gradient.

Although *intracellular* ATP may aid the transport of solutes through facilitating active transport, ingested ATP is *extracellular* and can thus not contribute to sodium absorption or facilitate secondary active transport.

Answer 12: MCQ

See *Medical Biochemistry at a Glance*, 3rd edn (**Transcription of DNA to make messenger RNA II**) and *Medical Sciences at a Glance* (**Gene expression**).

(b) The mechanism by which true tissue specificity of protein expression is achieved is alternative splicing. Operons are regulators of expression in bacteria and nematodes (d). Paternal and maternal DNA may be differentially expressed, especially in the case of X-inactivation in females, but this will not be tissue specific (e).

Answer 13: MCQ

See *Medical Biochemistry at a Glance*, 3rd edn (**Anaerobic glycolysis in red blood cells**) and *Medical Sciences at a Glance* (**Gas transport**).

(c) 2,3-Bisphosphoglycerate is an isomer of the glycolytic intermediate 1,3-bisphosphoglycerate. It is uniquely present in red blood cells, where it regulates the oxygen affinity of haemoglobin. Increased levels result in a decrease of haemoglobin's oxygen affinity.

Answer 14: True/False

See *Medical Biochemistry at a Glance*, 3rd edn (Oxidation of fatty acids and Diabetes mellitus) and *Medical Sciences at a Glance* (Fat as a fuel).

(a) **True**. Ketone body production occurs in the liver during fasting. A large amount of fatty acids returning from adipose tissue is oxidised by the liver, resulting in high levels of acetyl-CoA and NADH, more than is needed by the liver cells. The excess NADH, together with stimulation from glucagon, slows the citric acid cycle (NADH inhibits pyruvate dehydrogenase, isocitrate dehydrogenase and α-ketogluterate dehydrogenase) and thus acetyl-CoA levels rise and are channelled into ketone body production.

(b) **False**. Ketone bodies are water soluble and do not require the transport mechanisms used by fatty acids.

(c) **False**. The liver is the only significant site of ketone body synthesis, as only liver cells possess significant quantities of HMG CoA synthase.

(d) **False**. Ketone bodies are produced in mitochondria.

(e) **True**. Insulin will be therapeutic in this case. It will stimulate glucose absorption from the serum and end the pathological starvation. This will decrease ketone body *synthesis*.

Answer 15: MCQ

See *Medical Biochemistry at a Glance*, 3rd edn (Urea cycle and overview of amino acid catabolism).

(c) Ammonia, which is highly toxic, is metabolised by the urea cycle. This results in the formation of non-toxic urea that can be readily excreted in the urine. The rate-limiting step of the urea cycle is the creation of carbamoyl phosphate from ammonia and CO_2. The reaction is driven by the hydrolysis of two molecules of ATP.

Answer 16: EMQ

See *Medical Biochemistry at a Glance*, 3rd edn (Water-soluble vitamins I & II and Fat-soluble vitamins I–IV).

(1) **F**. Odd chain fatty acid breakdown requires vitamin B_{12} for the final step of odd chain fatty acid oxidation which involves the conversion of methylmalonyl-CoA to succinyl-CoA. The resulting accumulation of methylmalonic acid destabilises myelin and causes PNS and CNS degeneration.

(2) **G**. This classic picture of scurvy is rarely seen today. Vitamin C is required for proline hydroxylation, and without it, collagen uses its cross-links and tensile strength.

(3) **E**. Vitamin B_6 plays a role in transamination and the decarboxylation of glutamic acid to γ-aminobutyric acid (GABA). Isoniazid, which is part of the drug regimen for tuberculosis, causes depletion of this vitamin.

(4) **B**. Vitamin B_1, also known as thiamine, is often deficient in alcoholics and is required by key enzymes of carbohydrate metabolism and the pentose phosphate pathway. Red cell transketolase used to be an indirect test for thiamine.

(5) **D**. Niacin or vitamin B_3 is required for NAD and NADP, which are an important cellular energy currency. Deficiency results in pellagra with the features of diarrhoea, dermatitis and dementia (three 'Ds').

Answer 17: MCQ

See *Medical Genetics at a Glance*, 3rd edn (Aspects of dominance, Genomic inprinting and Dynamic mutation).

(c) Huntington's disease is most commonly discussed in the context of *anticipation*, which describes the increasingly earlier presentation of a disease with every subsequent generation that occurs with trinucleotide expansions. However, this is not what the vignette describes. The question describes the skipping of a generation by phenotype but not by genotype, suggesting variability in the expression of the genotype known as *variable penetrance*.

Answer 18: SAQ

See *Medical Sciences at a Glance* (General principles).

A simple example of a coupled reaction is the following (1).

$$glucose + ATP \xrightarrow{\ yields\ } glucose\ 6\ phosphate + ADP$$

The conversion of glucose to glucose-6-phosphate is thermodynamically unfavourable (2). However, by forming an intermediate with ATP, the conversion of glucose to glucose-6-phosphate becomes possible, being coupled to the energetically favourable hydrolysis of ATP to ADP (3).

Coupling has multiple advantages, such as the ability to use an energy currency such as ATP (4), as well as the ability to adjust the metabolic pathways to the current nutritional state (5).

Answer 19: MCQ

See *Medical Genetics at a Glance*, 3rd edn (The polymerase chain reaction).

(a) PCR doubles the amount of DNA available with each cycle, thus the square root needs to be taken. Division by 20 is necessary to account for the original viral particles, and finally 1 needs to be subtracted, as the initial DNA present counts as the initial step.

$$\sqrt{\frac{20000}{20}} - 1 = 9.$$

Answer 20: EMQ

See *Medical Genetics at a Glance*, 3rd edn (Sex chromosome aneuploidies and Autosomal aneuploidies) and *Medical Sciences at a Glance* (Medical genetics).

(1) **E**. Two Barr bodies in a woman suggest the karyotype XXX (triple X syndrome), which has not been associated with any definite phenotypic abnormalities, although studies have raised possible associations. In a male, having any number of Barr bodies is characteristic of Klinefelter syndrome.

(2) **F**. Friedreich ataxia is caused by GAA triplet expansion in the frataxin gene that causes its inactivation. It causes a variety of neurological signs and symptoms and becomes apparent during childhood or early adolescence.

(3) **H**. The scenario is not unusual for individuals with Turner syndrome, who frequently are not diagnosed with their condition until adulthood. The karyotype would show only one X chromosome.

(4) **D**. Edwards syndrome is a rare trisomy which often results in prenatal death. It has a poor prognosis of 1–2 years for live births. Patau syndrome is due to trisomy 13.

(5) **G**. The answer suggests a trinucleotide repeat disorder inherited on the X chromosome (maternal uncle suggests X-linked recessive inheritance). The features described in the vignette point to Kennedy disease, also known as spinobulbar muscular atrophy. Fragile X syndrome is characterised by a CGG expansion and causes mental retardation and characteristic features from birth.

Answer 21: SAQ
See *Medical Biochemistry at a Glance*, 3rd edn (**What happens when protons or electrons leak from the respiratory chain?**) and *Medical Sciences at a Glance* (**Central metabolic pathways**).
After the addition of 300 nmol of ADP, the O_2 concentration falls from 0.2 to 0.1 mM. A drop in 0.1 mM means that 200 nmol of O molecules were consumed. Thus the ATP:O ratio is 1.5.

In the second experiment nothing happens after the addition of ADP at time point 1. This could be due to inhibition of ATP synthesis or the electron transport chain. The addition of an uncoupler still results in rapid oxygen consumption, suggesting that the electron transport chain is working, and thus X must be an inhibitor of ATP formation.

Answer 22: MCQ
See *Medical Biochemistry at a Glance*, 3rd edn (**Metabolism of amino acids and porphyrins**) and *Medical Sciences at a Glance* (**Amino acid metabolism**).
(c) Although the majority of muscle ammonium is transported to the liver via the alanine-glucose shuttle, some ammonium is incorporated into glutamine. Glutaminase is found in the liver and kidneys, but the renal excretion of ammonium ions is only significant in acidosis.

Answer 23: True/False
See *Medical Biochemistry at a Glance*, 3rd edn (**Comparison of DNA replication, DNA transcription and protein synthesis in eukaryotes and prokaryotes**).
(a) **False**. 40S subunits form *eukaryotic* ribosomes. *Prokaryotic* ribosomes have 30S and 50S subunits.
(b) **True**. The Shine–Dalgarno sequence (AGGAGG) is only found in prokaryotes. It is found 8 base pairs upstream of the AUG start codon.
(c) **True**. The ρ factor is one of the prokaryotic mechanisms for termination of transcription. It attaches to the mRNA that is being synthesised and moves along the mRNA towards RNA polymerase to terminate its action.
(d) **False**. Reverse transcriptase is found in retroviruses, not bacteria.
(e) **True**. Although there are no such antibiotics on the market, this is a potential drug target. In practice, it has not been possible to create prokaryote-specific nucleoside analogues. Many of the currently used antiretroviral drugs are, however, nucleoside analogues.

Answer 24: MCQ
See *Medical Biochemistry at a Glance*, 3rd edn (**HDL metabolism**) and *Medical Sciences at a Glance* (**Cardiovascular pathophysiology**).
(b) As HDL takes up cholesterol, it immediately esterifies it by activating lecithin-cholesterol acyltransferase (LCAT). The main functions of HDL include reverse cholesterol transport (c); it also serves as a reservoir for Apo C-II and Apo E (a). The cholesterol accumulated by HDL is delivered to the liver (d). Diets high in cholesterol, unsaturated and trans fatty acid, which are abundant in fast food, result in a *high LDL* and *low HDL* (e).

Answer 25: MCQ
See *Medical Biochemistry at a Glance*, 3rd edn (**Steroid hormones**) and *Medical Sciences at a Glance* (**Adrenal gland and steroid hormones**).
(b) 17-α-Hydroxylase allows the synthesis of both corticosteroids and sex hormones from pregnenolone and progesterone. However, it does not inhibit the mineralocorticoid pathway, resulting in overproduction of mineralocorticoids and thus hypertension. There is also feminisation due to the lack of testosterone and hypocortisolism.

Both 21α- and 11β-hydroxylase deficiencies result in loss of the glucocorticoid and mineralocorticoid pathways (c, d). They thus overproduce sex steroids, leading to virilisation, and both feature hypocortisolism. However, because 11β-hydroxylase is later in the pathway, 11-deoxycorticosterone, an effective mineralocorticoid, is produced with this deficiency, resulting in hypertension.

Answer 26: SAQ
See *Medical Biochemistry at a Glance*, 3rd edn (**Oxidation of fatty acids**) and *Medical Sciences at a Glance* (**Fat as a fuel**).
Fatty acid oxidation leads to the production of ATP, NADH and acetyl-CoA (1). Acetyl-CoA can enter the citric acid cycle (2), just like acetyl-CoA derived from glycolysis. However, both carbons provided by acetyl-CoA are converted to CO_2 (3). Oxaloacetate can be exported from mitochondria and converted to glucose in the liver (4). This, however, would deplete the pool of ketoacids required for the normal function of the citric acid cycle (5).

Similarly citrate can also be exported into the cytosol (4), but in the cytosol it is broken down to acetyl-CoA and oxaloacetate, the latter of which needs to return to the mitochondria to avoid depletion of the citric acid cycle (5).

Answer 27: MCQ
See *Medical Biochemistry at a Glance*, 3rd edn (**Anaerobic glycolysis in red blood cells**) and *Medical Sciences at a Glance* (**Gas transport**).
(d) At high altitude, oxygen is sparse and thus partial pressures of oxygen are lower. The body adapts by *decreasing* the oxygen affinity of haemoglobin via 2,3-BPG (right shift of the curve). This might sound counterintuitive, but what it does is facilitate the release of oxygen in the tissues. A left shift of the curve (b) occurs when BPG levels are low or if the pH rises or CO_2 concentrations fall, indicating good tissue oxygenation. Graph (e) shows a lowered oxygen saturation and this may occur in the presence of a competitive inhibitor, such as carbon monoxide. Graph (a) shows a binding curve without co-operativity, and is usually seen in myoglobin. Haemoglobin has the characteristic S shape that results from co-operative binding. Graph (c) shows no change.

Answer 28: True/False
See *Medical Biochemistry at a Glance*, 3rd edn (**Insulin signal transduction**) and *Medical Sciences at a Glance* (**Carbohydrates**).
(a) **True**. During fasting, glucagon signalling through a cAMP-dependent pathway will result in phosphorylation of glycogen synthase by cAMP-dependent protein kinase A. The phosphorylated enzyme is inactive.

(b) **True**. Glycogen synthase, which makes α(1→4) bonds, cannot commence glycogen synthesis *de novo*. If glycogen stores are depleted, the tyrosine of glycogenin serves as the starting point for glycogen synthesis.

(c) **False**. UDP-glucose, an activated form of glucose, is the substrate for glycogen synthase.

(d) **False**. Insulin is a hormone that does not penetrate into cells and does not modulate the activity of glycogen synthase directly. It binds to a tyrosine kinase, which initiates a signalling cascade that increases glycogen synthesis.

(e) **False**. Glycogen synthase forms α(1→4) bonds.

Answer 29: MCQ

See *Medical Biochemistry at a Glance*, 3rd edn (Transcription of DNA to make messenger RNA (II)) and *Medical Sciences at a Glance* (Gene expression).

(b) snRNPs, or small nuclear ribonucleic particles, are RNA–protein complexes that are important in the formation of splice-osomes and thus post-transcriptional modification.

Answer 30: EMQ

See *Medical Biochemistry at a Glance*, 3rd edn (Urea cycle and Amino acid disorders) and *Medical Sciences at a Glance* (Amino acid metabolism).

(1) **A**. Muscle, in contrast to most other tissues, excretes its ammonia in the form of alanine. Alanine is then transported to the liver where it is deaminated, and the resulting pyruvate is metabolised to glucose via gluconeogenesis. The glucose then returns to the muscle to provide energy via glycolysis – this is known as the glucose–alanine cycle.

(2) **E**. Glutamine serves as a non-toxic storage form of ammonia. It is synthesised in all tissues, and can be degraded to release free ammonia by the liver or the kidneys. Excretion of ammonia by kidneys is dependent on the acid–base equilibrium and only ever significant in acidosis.

(3) **I**. Ornithine is not one of the 20 amino acids coded for by DNA and this is not used for protein synthesis. It is found in the urea cycle.

(4) **I**. Carbamoyl phosphate synthetase combines ammonia and carbon dioxide to form carbamoyl phosphate, which is combined with ornithine to form citrulline. The lack of carbamoyl phosphate arrests this reaction that is catalysed by ornithine transcarbamylase and results in the accumulation of ornithine. Ornithine also accumulates in ornithine transcarbamylase deficiency.

(5) **I**. Cystine, ornithine, lysine and arginine (mnemonic: COLA) use the same transport mechanism for reabsorption of these amino acids from the proximal tubule. Although it is cystinuria that causes most problems by stone formation, deficiency of the transport system affects the other amino acids as well, resulting in their increased excretion. However, they are more soluble and can also use an alternative transport system not available to cystine, and thus do not cause disease.

4 Biochemistry and genetics exam 2

Questions

Question 1: MCQ

A sprinter's blood is taken immediately after a 200 metre run and shows a high content of lactic acid. Increased levels of which of the following drive the production of lactic acid in a muscle cell during sprint?

(a) NADP
(b) Glucose
(c) NADH
(d) ATP
(e) High CO_2

Question 2: True/False

You work as a geneticist and are looking at karyotypes. Which of the following statements are true?

(a) In a child with Down syndrome, who has a karyotype with 46 chromosomes, the illness has arisen due to a balanced translocation between two acrocentric chromosomes in one of his parents.
(b) A balanced translocation usually does not cause phenotypic changes in the first generation it occurs in.
(c) Chromosomal translocations during gametogenesis occur due to non-disjunction.
(d) The Philadelphia chromosome is an example of an unbalanced translocation.
(e) Balanced translocations can give rise to unbalanced translocations in offspring.

Question 3: MCQ

An athlete's plasma insulin level rises steeply after the ingestion of a carbonated drink. Insulin action will result in the translocation of which molecule to the cell surface of muscle cells?

(a) GLUT1
(b) GLUT2
(c) GLUT3
(d) GLUT4
(e) GLUT5

Question 4: SAQ (5 points)

A microbiologist investigates a bacterial plasmid that confers methicillin resistance. To further analyse the plasmid, he subjects the isolated plasmid to digestion by endonucleases. The following endonucleases are used and the results are seen using agarose gel electrophoresis (Figure 4.1). The first row includes EcoRI, the second includes BamHI, the third includes HndII, the fourth includes EcoRI and BamHI, the fifth includes EcoRI and HndII and the sixth includes BamHI and HndII.

Draw a restriction map for the above plasmid. The seventh row includes plasmid without any endonucleases – what is the explanation for its size? What is the purpose of the eighth row?

Question 5: MCQ

A 45-year-old alcoholic presents with a decreased conscious state. He has increased levels of serum ammonia which cannot be metabolised by the damaged liver. Which *one* of the following is true about the metabolism of ammonia?

(a) Ammonia is converted to urea by transamination.
(b) The reactions that incorporate ammonia into the urea cycle occur in the mitochondrial membrane.
(c) The build-up of ammonia will lower the pH of the blood.
(d) Ammonia cannot be excreted by the kidney, unless it is first incorporated into urea in the liver.
(e) A significant proportion of ammonia is produced by intestinal bacteria which carry urease.

Question 6: MCQ

A young child with cystic fibrosis is diagnosed with a vitamin deficiency of a fat-soluble vitamin. Which of the following is most probably deficient?

(a) Retinol (vitamin A)
(b) Riboflavin (vitamin B_2)
(c) Niacin (vitamin B_3)

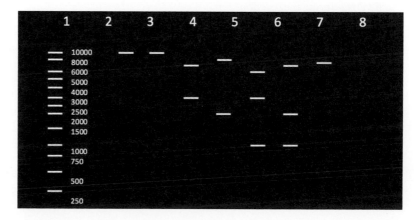

Figure 4.1 Results from the agarose electrophoresis experiment.

Medical Sciences at a Glance: Practice Workbook, First Edition. Jakub Scaber, Faisal Rahman and Peter Abrahams. © 2014 John Wiley & Sons, Ltd. **33**

(d) Ascorbic acid (vitamin C)

(e) Biotin (vitamin H)

Question 7: EMQ

A VLDL

B HDL

C Non-esterified fatty acids

D Ketone bodies

E Phospholipids

F Chylomicrons

G LDL

H Triacylglycerides

I Cholesterol

For each question below, choose the correct option from the list above.

(1) A 26-year-old man sees his GP for yellow lesions on his elbows and knees. A blood test shows elevated triglycerides, which are carried by an envelope of phospholipid that is characterised by the presence of apolipoprotein B-48. What are these particles called?

(2) A 44-year-old obese lady with a gallstone in the common bile duct has fatty stools. A component of bile responsible for emulsification of fat no longer reaches the gut. What is this component synthesized from?

(3) A GP analyses the results of a lipid screen. High levels of which of the above have a favourable effect on cardiovascular health?

(4) Which of the above provides the major energy supply of the brain during fasting?

(5) Which of the above provides 80% of the heart's energy requirement?

Question 8: True/False

An infant with severe developmental delay, lactic acidosis and motor weakness is found to have Leigh syndrome. Underlying this condition is a mutation in the gene coding for succinate dehydrogenase which catalyses the conversion of succinate to fumarate. Malonate is a competitive inhibitor of succinate dehydrogenase.

(a) A fall in the concentration of malonate will raise the K_m of succinate dehydrogenase.

(b) A rise in the concentration of malonate will decrease the V_{max} of succinate dehydrogenase.

(c) The lactic acidosis is caused by increased lactic acid production secondary to inhibition of the TCA cycle.

(d) The reaction is irreversible because FAD is reduced to FADH2 during the reaction.

(e) Succinate dehydrogenase is part of the electron transport chain.

Question 9: MCQ

When investigating the effect of a poison on the electron transport chain in your laboratory, you find that complexes I, II and III are in their reduced state, but cytochrome c and complex IV are oxidised. Which poison can inhibit the electron transport chain to give this result?

(a) Amytal

(b) Antimycin A

(c) Carbon monoxide

(d) Dinitrophenol

(e) Rotenone

Question 10: SAQ (5 points)

During the fasting state glucagon triggers the release of glucose from the liver. What are the steps in this signalling cascade and why are there so many?

Question 11: MCQ

During a routine blood test a 45-year-old woman is found to have mild anaemia with a raised unconjugated bilirubin. She is finally diagnosed with pyruvate kinase deficiency. This is further investigated in the laboratory and her level of decreased pyruvate kinase function is caused by an inability to respond to the main activator of pyruvate kinase. What molecule activates pyruvate kinase?

(a) Glucose

(b) Glucose-6-phosphate

(c) ATP

(d) Fructose 1,6-bisphosphate

(e) Lactate

Question 12: EMQ

A DNA cloning

B Polymerase chain reaction (PCR)

C Western blotting

D Northern blotting

E Southern blotting

F DNA sequencing

G Fluorescence *in situ* hybridisation (FISH)

H Polyacrylamide gel electrophoresis (SDS-PAGE)

I Agarose gel electrophoresis

For each question below, choose the correct option from the list above.

(1) An autopsy is performed on a 45-year-old man who suffered from early-onset dementia. Creutzfeldt–Jakob disease is suspected. The disease is caused by a misfolded protein that is resistant to pretreatment with digestive enzymes. In normal individuals the protein is digested into smaller fragments. Which technique should be used to detect the difference between the normal and misfolded proteins?

(2) A piece of hair is found at a crime scene. The DNA is extracted and short tandem repeat regions that are characteristic of a particular individual are amplified using the usual techniques. What technique will be used to visualise and compare the amplified material?

(3) Scientists identify an unknown restriction fragment length polymorphism that is closely linked to an inherited condition. What technique should they use to obtain enough copies for sequencing?

(4) A couple undergoing *in vitro* fertilisation request preimplantation diagnosis for the most common genetic conditions. Which of the above techniques should be used to detect Down syndrome in a single embryonal cell obtained from an eight-cell morula?

(5) A Cypriot immigrant wants to know if she is a carrier for Duchenne muscular dystrophy, a disease that runs in her families. What technique will be used to determine this?

Question 13: MCQ

Celiac disease is a condition affecting the bowel by immune-mediated damage to the bowel wall. The wall damage leads to malabsorption

due to loss of an important enzyme on the brush border. What is the name of this enzyme, which activates the zymogens released from the pancreas?
(a) Carboxypeptidase
(b) Elastase
(c) Enteropeptidase
(d) Lipase
(e) Trypsin

Question 14: EMQ

A DNA polymerase α
B DNA polymerase γ
C DNA polymerase δ
D Telomerase
E Helicase
F Origin recognition complex
G Topoisomerase I
H Topoisomerase II
I DnaA protein
J Single-stranded binding protein
K DNA polymerase I
L DNA polymerase III
M Ligase

For each question below, choose the correct option from the list above.
(1) Aphidicolin is a compound that arrests bacterial DNA synthesis in the S phase by inhibiting the enzyme that replaces RNA primers with DNA. Which of the above fits this explanation?
(2) Activation of this enzyme immortalises cancer cells and is found in 90% of all human tumours.
(3) Retinoblastoma protein is a tumour suppressor gene that has been shown to control the initiation of DNA synthesis in human eukaryotes. Which of the above is thus under control by retinoblastoma?
(4) Ciprofloxacin is an antibacterial that inhibits an enzyme, which prevents supercoiling and has the ability to introduce negative supercoils to facilitate replication.
(5) Incorporation of matching overlapping DNA strands into vectors is an important step in recombinant DNA technology. Which enzyme will form covalent bonds between 3' hydroxyl and 5' phosphate backbones?

Question 15: MCQ

A 35-year-old woman with a BMI of 29 decides to embark on a prolonged, absolutely fat-free diet. Which of the following will her body not be able to synthesise or obtain from her diet?
(a) Prostaglandins
(b) Bile acids
(c) Phospholipids
(d) Ketones
(e) Oestrogen

Question 16: True/False

A researcher finds an activating mutation in Akt1 in breast, colo-rectal and ovarian cancer. Which of the following statements about Akt, also known as protein kinase B, are true?
(a) Akt promotes apoptosis through the activation of bad.
(b) When active, Akt is closely associated with the cell membrane.

(c) Akt requires high levels of the second messenger cAMP for function.
(d) Akt is a G-protein.
(e) Activation of Akt promotes cellular proliferation through the inhibition of GSK3, which results in the release of the transcription factor β-catenin.

Question 17: MCQ

A 7-year-old child is investigated for progressive proximal muscle weakness. A muscle biopsy shows numerous fat droplets. Which micronutrient is necessary for the transport of fatty acids into mitochondria?
(a) Biotin
(b) Niacin
(c) Carnitine
(d) Adenosine
(e) Vitamin B_{12}

Question 18: SAQ (5 points)

A 35-year-old woman with a history of depression is brought to the hospital with severe recurrent hypoglycaemia. How would you distinguish between a self-inflicted hypoglycaemia due to injection of synthetic insulin and an overproduction of insulin by a tumour (insulinoma)?

Question 19: MCQ

A 24-year-old man is on the intensive care unit with meningitis. His blood lactate concentration is 6 mmol/L, and the pK_a of lactic acid is 3.9. His blood pH is 6.9. What concentration of lactic acid will be circulating in the acid (HA) form?
(a) 6 μmol/L
(b) 60 μmol/L
(c) 750 μmol/L
(d) 5940 μmol/L
(e) 5994 μmol/L

Question 20: EMQ

A Primary structure
B Secondary structure
C Hydrophobic interactions
D Supersecondary structure
E Van der Waals interactions
F Tertiary structure
G Quaternary structure

For each statement below, choose the correct option from the list above.
(1) C-myc is an important proto-oncogene, and upregulation is commonly found in lung cancer cells. To bind DNA, it relies on a helix-loop-helix domain. This is an example of …
(2) Co-operative binding of oxygen by haemoglobin is a feature of its …
(3) The disulphide bonds of ribonuclease stabilise its …
(4) Keratin is a structural protein whose structure is almost entirely α-helical. This is an example of …
(5) During septic shock, proteins in the body are more susceptible to denaturation. Which of the above is least likely to be altered by denaturation?

Question 21: MCQ

A couple attends the genetic clinic. The man has cystic fibrosis while the woman is homozygous for the wild-type gene. They already have a daughter who is still a child, and has not been tested. They want to know the theoretical chances of passing on the disease to their grandchildren. If the population is assumed to be in equilibrium, and the prevalence of the disease is 1/2500, what is the chance that a grandchild will have the disease?

(a) 1/4
(b) 1/12
(c) 1/25
(d) 1/50
(e) 1/100

Question 22: SAQ (5 points)

A patient eats a fatty meal. Outline how intestinal absorption of triglyceride is achieved. How does absorption of short and medium chain fatty acids differ?

Question 23: MCQ

A long distance runner is approaching the finish line. How does muscle contraction affect myocyte metabolism? Please select *one* answer.

(a) Muscle contraction does not affect myocyte metabolism directly.
(b) Calcium release from the smooth endoplasmic reticulum to the cytoplasm stimulates glycogenolysis and gluconeogenesis.
(c) Calcium release from the smooth endoplasmic reticulum to the cytoplasm inhibits the citric acid cycle.
(d) Calcium release from the smooth endoplasmic reticulum to the cytoplasm stimulates glycogen phosphorylase and citric acid cycle enzymes.
(e) Calcium causes activation of its substrates by direct allostery.

Question 24: True/False

A 65-year-old woman visits her GP with symptoms of painless progressive jaundice and pale stools. She is eventually diagnosed with obstruction of the common bile duct by a pancreatic tumour. Which of the following statements about bile are true?

(a) Bile salts give the stool its colour.
(b) Bile contains important enzymes that are required for the digestion of lipids.
(c) Bile salts are synthesised in the liver.
(d) Bile salts emulsify fats in the intestine and form chylomicrons.
(e) The liver will adapt to the obstruction by producing less conjugated bilirubin.

Question 25: MCQ

A woman suffering from systemic lupus erythematosus has antibodies to snRNPs. Which process will be affected?

(a) DNA repair
(b) RNA synthesis
(c) Splicing
(d) Phagocytosis
(e) Protein degradation

Question 26: True/False

A 24-year-old student from Italy presents with shortness of breath following a course of trimethoprim-sulfamethoxazole. He is found to be anaemic and is diagnosed with glucose-6-phosphate dehydrogenase (G6PD) deficiency. G6PD is part of a pathway which is involved in which of the following?

(a) Amino acid synthesis
(b) Fatty acid biosynthesis
(c) Oxidative phosphorylation
(d) Reduction of reactive oxygen species
(e) DNA synthesis

Question 27: EMQ

A Repressor of enzyme synthesis
B Inducer of enzyme synthesis
C Competitive inhibitor
D Non-competitive inhibitor
E Irreversible inhibitor
F Homotropic inhibitor
G Heterotropic inhibitor
H Allosteric activator

For each question below, choose the correct option from the list above.

(1) Dihydrofolate reductase is an enzyme that catalyses the reaction from dihydrofolate to tetrahydrofolate. After adding methotrexate, an antineoplastic and immunosuppressant that acts on this enzyme, the K_m of the enzyme apparently increases, while the V_{max} remains constant. What best describes methotrexate?
(2) Phosphofructokinase-1 regulates the committed step of glycolysis and is thus under tight regulation. What best describes the role of ATP with regard to PFK-1?
(3) Citrate concentrations also regulate phosphofructokinase. How is the action of citrate on phosphofructokinase-1 best described?
(4) Angiotensin converting enzyme catalyses the reaction from angiotensin I to angiotensin II. In the presence of ramipril, the Limeweaver–Burk plot changes as follows: the intercept with the Y axis remains constant, whereas the intercept with the X axis becomes more positive. What best describes the action of ramipril?
(5) Cyclo-oxygenase converts arachidonic acid to prostaglandin H2. After adding aspirin, the V_{max} of the enzyme markedly drops. After washing out the drug, the decrease in V_{max} is still seen. How does aspirin affect cyclo-oxygenase?

Question 28: MCQ

A young woman requires a blood transfusion and is found to be in blood group A. This statement describes her blood:

(a) character
(b) gene
(c) allele
(d) genotype
(e) phenotype

Question 29: SAQ (5 points)

In nucleotide repeat disorders such as fragile X, why are three nucleotides repeated rather than two or four?

Question 30: MCQ

A 24-year-old man is brought to A&E with abdominal pain. He is found to have alcoholic hepatitis. When the nurse checks his blood glucose (BM) it is only 1.4 mmol/L. What is the cause for this?

(a) Alcohol inhibits the action of glucagon.
(b) Alcohol stimulates the release of insulin.
(c) Alcohol inhibits gluconeogenesis in the liver.
(d) Alcohol inhibits the production of lactic acid.
(e) Alcohol inhibits the respiratory chain.

Answer 1: MCQ

See *Medical Biochemistry at a Glance*, 3rd edn (**Anaerobic oxidation of glucose by glycolysis to form ATP and lactate**) and *Medical Sciences at a Glance* (**Glucose as a fuel**).

(c) During a sprint the NADH production by glycolysis (glyceraldehyde 3-phosphate dehydrogenase) exceeds the oxidative capacity of the electron transport chain. The high concentration of NADH results in the reduction of pyruvate to lactate and concomitant oxidation of NADH to NAD⁺. The other compounds do not affect lactate production.

Answer 2: True/False

See *Medical Genetics at a Glance*, 2nd edn (**Chromosome structural abnormalities and Chromosome structural abnormalities, clinical examples**) and *Medical Sciences at a Glance* (**Medical genetics**).

(a) **True**. Robertsonian translocations are quasi-balanced translocations that result in the creation of a single chromosome from two acrocentric (with almost non-existent short arms) chromosomes. The short arms are lost, and instead a large chromosome with two long arms is created, resulting in 45 chromosomes in the parent. When such a translocation involving chromosome 21 is passed on, it may result in Down syndrome with a numerically normal complement of chromosomes, as the new chromosome will carry a third copy of the genes present on chromosome 21.

(b) **True**. A balanced translocation results in an even exchange between two chromosomes and most commonly does not result in any phenotypic changes in the generation that carries the translocation. However, it may result in an unbalanced translocation in the following generation.

(c) **False**. Translocations commonly occur during oogenesis as oocytes spend a long time in prophase I. The mechanism is likely to include the chance joining of the short arms or centromeres of two acrocentric chromosomes, and does not occur during the metaphase/anaphase transition like nondisjunction would do.

(d) **False**. The Philadelphia chromosome results in the oncogenic BCR-ABL gene fusion that leads to overexpression of a tyrosine kinase. However, no genetic material is lost or gained, thus the translocation is balanced.

(e) **True**. Balanced translocations usually occur in the parent generation. Because no information is lost or gained, the parent has an apparently normal genome. However, during gametogenesis this results in two uneven gametes with excess of some genetic information and surplus of other genes. This leads to an unbalanced translocation in the offspring.

Answer 3: MCQ

See *Medical Biochemistry at a Glance*, 3rd edn (**Regulation of glycolysis and Krebs cycle**) and *Medical Sciences at a Glance* (**Glucose as a fuel**).

(d) The glucose transporter type 4 (GLUT4) is found in adipose cells and striated muscle and is translocated to the cell membrane in response to insulin signalling. It facilitates the influx of glucose into these cells during the fed state. None of the other transporters is insulin dependent. GLUT2 is the high-capacity but low-affinity isoform found in the liver, renal tubules and pancreatic β cells. GLUT1 regulates basal glucose uptake by all cells and GLUT3 is found in neurons. GLUT5 is a fructose transporter.

Answer 4: SAQ

See *Medical Genetics at a Glance*, 3rd edn (**DNA hybridization-based analysis systems**) and *Medical Sciences at a Glance* (**Principles of molecular genetics**) (5 points).

(3 points for restriction map)

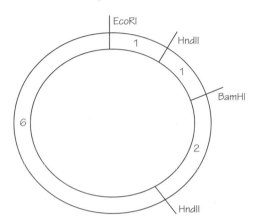

Figure 4.2 Restriction map based on the plasmid endonucleases seen on the electrophoresis gel. Numbers on restriction map indicate size of fragments in kilobases.

Because the uncut plasmids are supercoiled, they travel faster through the gel than the linear plasmids in rows 1 and 2, resulting in an apparent decrease in size (4). The final row probably represents a negative control run with distilled water to exclude any contamination in the gel (5) (Figure 4.2).

Answer 5: MCQ

See *Medical Biochemistry at a Glance*, 3rd edn (**Urea cycle**) and *Medical Sciences at a Glance* (**Amino acid metabolism**).

(e) The cleavage of urea by intestinal bacteria is an important contributor to the hyperammonaemia seen in hepatic encephalopathy. Reduction of this production by use of laxatives and antibiotics is an important treatment modality. Transamination shuttles the ammonia groups between sugar backbones but cannot incorporate free ammonia (a). Two amino groups are incorporated into the urea cycle: the first is provided by the incorporation of aspartate in the cytosol. A free ammonium ion is incorporated into carbamoyl phosphate in the mitochondrial matrix, not its membrane (b). Ammonia is a weak base, so will increase the pH of blood and plays an important role in acid–base regulation (c). A proportion of ammonia is excreted directly by the kidneys by hydrolysis of ammonia by the enzyme glutaminase (d).

Answer 6: MCQ

See *Medical Biochemistry at a Glance*, 3rd edn (**Fat-soluble vitamins**) and *Medical Sciences at a Glance* (**The liver**).

(a) Cystic fibrosis is caused by a genetic mutation in a chloride transporter, which results in thickened viscous secretions. This causes bronchiectasis in the lungs but it also manifests by obstruction of the pancreatic ducts by viscous pancreatic secretions, that cannot provide enough lipase for absorption of lipids, including fat-soluble vitamins, which are A, D, E and K.

Answer 7: EMQ
See *Medical Biochemistry at a Glance*, 3rd edn (Absorption and disposal of dietary triacylglycerols, HDL metabolism, VLDL and LDL metabolism and Metabolism of carbohydrate to cholesterol).
(1) **F**. Chylomicrons are synthesised in the large intestine and contain apolipoprotein B-48. The described disease is type I hyperlipoproteinaemia, caused by decreased lipoprotein lipase function and resulting in chylomicronaemia.
(2) **I**. Bile salts are made from cholesterol, which is modified in a multistep process and conjugated to glycine or taurine.
(3) **B**. HDL cholesterol is also known as 'good cholesterol'. Levels above 1 mmol/L (40 mg/dL) correlate well with reduced cardiovascular mortality.
(4) **D**. Ketone bodies provide the bulk of the energy supply to the brain during fasting.
(5) **C**. Non-esterified fatty acids provide the major energy source to the heart, which relies on oxidative phosphorylation. The NADH is provided by products of fatty acid degradation.

Answer 8: True/False
See *Medical Biochemistry at a Glance*, 3rd edn (Aerobic production of ATP) and *Medical Sciences at a Glance* (Central metabolic pathways).
(a) **True**. The K_m is apparently raised in the presence of a competitive inhibitor.
(b) **False**. Competitive inhibition does not affect V_{max}.
(c) **True**. Cytosolic NADH produced by glycolysis will accumulate and drive the production of lactic acid. Cytosolic NADH can be used to fuel oxidative phosphorylation but relies on the citric acid cycle to do this, as transport into the mitochondria occurs via the malate–aspartate shuttle.
(d) **False**. The fact that a reaction results in reduction of a co-factor does not make it irreversible. In truly irreversible reactions, one of the products exits the reacting system, making the reverse reaction impossible. Reactions with large free energy changes are also called irreversible, as the equilibrium constant is large, so that the products never reach equilibrium under physiological conditions. In the citric acid cycle, these reactions are catalysed by the enzymes citrate synthase, isocitrate dehydrogenase and α-ketogluterate dehydrogenase.
(e) **True**. Succinate dehydrogenase is best known as part of the Krebs cycle but is also known as complex II of the electron transport chain, and is bound to the inner mitochondrial membrane. FAD, the electron acceptor, is known as co-enzyme Q.

Answer 9: MCQ
See *Medical Biochemistry at a Glance*, 3rd edn (Biosynthesis of ATP) and *Medical Sciences at a Glance* (Central metabolic pathways).
(b) Antimicin A inhibits the transfer of electrons from complex III to cytochrome c; thus complex III is reduced but cytochrome c remains oxidised. The remaining poisons inhibit the electron transport chain at different points: amytal and rotenone inhibit the passing on of electrons from complex I, and carbon monoxide inhibits transfer of electrons from complex IV to oxygen. Dinitrophenol does not inhibit the electron transport chain and instead uncouples ATP synthesis from the electron transport chain by dissipating the gradient created by the electron transport chain.

Answer 10: SAQ
See *Medical Biochemistry at a Glance*, 3rd edn (Regulation of glycogen metabolism).
(1) Glucagon binds to its receptor which activates a G-protein.
(2) G-protein activates adenylyl cyclase which causes a rise in cAMP.
(3) cAMP activates cAMP-dependent protein kinase.
(4) cAMP-dependent protein kinase activates glycogen phosphorylase kinase.
(5) Glycogen phosphorylase kinase activates glycogen phosphorylase.

These five steps all allow amplification of the signal – few hormone molecules activate a large number of glycogen phosphorylase molecules that then degrade glycogen.

Answer 11: MCQ
See *Medical Biochemistry at a Glance*, 3rd edn (Regulation of glycolysis and Krebs cycle).
(d) Pyruvate kinase catalyses the reaction from phosphoenolpyruvate to pyruvate. ATP is formed by this reaction, and decreased levels of ADP may inhibit the enzyme. Fructose 1,6-bisphosphate is an allosteric activator of pyruvate kinase, and signals increased glycolysis. A mutation that affects the site of binding of fructose 1,6-bisphosphate is among the reasons for pyruvate kinase deficiency. The remaining choices in this question do not affect pyruvate kinase activity directly.

Answer 12: EMQ
See *Medical Genetics at a Glance*, 3rd edn (DNA hybridization-based analysis systems, The polymerase chain reaction, Physical gene mapping and DNA sequencing) or *Medical Sciences at a Glance* (Principles of molecular genetics).
(1) **C**. Western blotting is the technique used to analyse proteins. It consists of two steps: initially proteins are separated by size using SDS-PAGE electrophoresis, followed by transfer onto a nitrocellulose membrane for identification using radiolabelling.
(2) **I**. Amplification of tandem repeat regions in criminology is done by PCR. However, the particles then need to be run through an agarose gel to determine their sizes and make a comparison – this spatially resolves the particles. Southern blotting involves transfer of the DNA onto a membrane and application of a probe for identification, but this is not needed as the sample has undergone probe-dependent amplification and any irrelevant DNA will be negligible. SDS-PAGE is used for proteins.
(3) **A**. The key here is that the sequence of the RFLP is unknown, requiring laborious DNA cloning to provide enough copies of DNA for sequencing. The sequence would have to be known to design primers for PCR.

(4) **G.** Fluorescent *in situ* hybridisation is an inexpensive, quick and effective method that is used to test a range of genetic conditions. After isolation of the chromosomes, a fluorescent marker for chromosome 21 is applied and the number of chromosomes with the fluorescent marker is counted. If there are three signals then Down syndrome can be diagnosed.

(5) **F.** DNA sequencing has become more available for a number of known diseases. Sequencing the patient's dystrophin gene will give the best answer.

Answer 13: MCQ

See *Medical Sciences at a Glance* (Lower GI physiology).

(c) Enteropeptidase is the brush border enzyme that initiates the activation of peptidases from zymogens secreted by the pancreas. Once a small amount of trypsin is formed from trypsinogen, it takes over as it cleaves both trypsinogen and other zymogens more effectively.

Answer 14: EMQ

See *Medical Biochemistry at a Glance*, 3rd edn (Structure of DNA, Replication of DNA I & II and Comparison of DNA replication, DNA transcription and protein synthesis in prokaryotes and eukaryotes) and *Medical Sciences at a Glance* (DNA and RNA).

(1) **K.** Aphidicolin is mainly used in experimental settings. It inhibits the replacement of RNA primers in the lagging strand in bacteria, a task carried out by DNA polymerase I. It has a 5' to 3' DNA polymerase as well as proofreading activity, but is considerably slower than DNA polymerase III. Aphidicolin also inhibits eukaryotic polymerases α and δ.

(2) **D.** Telomerase is required for 'immortality' of cell lines, as it prevents the destabilisation of the genome by shortening of telomeres with each successive replication.

(3) **F.** The origin recognition complex is required for initiation of transcription. Its activation is dependent on the G_1 checkpoint, which is under tight control. One of the regulators of the G_1 checkpoint is retinoblastoma which, when phosphorylated, releases the transcription factor E2F, resulting in progression to S phase.

(4) **H.** Fluoroquinolones, including ciprofloxacin, are inhibitors of prokaryotic topoisomerase II. Only type II topoisomerase, also known as DNA gyrase, nicks and then re-anneals both strands of DNA and is thus able to introduce negative supercoils into relaxed circular bacterial DNA.

(5) **M.** DNA ligase fixes single-stranded discontinuities in double-stranded DNA; an application of this is the annealing of 'sticky' ends in recombinant DNA technology.

Answer 15: MCQ

See *Medical Biochemistry at a Glance*, 3rd edn (Structure of lipids) or *Medical Sciences at a Glance* (Lipids).

(a) All but the essential fatty acids (linoleic acid and linolenic acid) can be synthesised from proteins and carbohydrates through fatty acid biosynthesis. Essential fatty acids are required for the synthesis of eicosanoids, biologically active lipids, such as prostaglandins, prostacyclins and leukotrienes. (Note: EPA and DHA can be synthesised from linolenic acid.)

Answer 16: True/False

See *Medical Biochemistry at a Glance*, 3rd edn (Insulin signal transduction and diabetes mellitus and The cell cycle).

(a) **False.** Akt is an inhibitor of bad, which is a pro-apoptotic protein. The Akt/PKB pathway is activated in response to growth signals, and inhibits apoptosis through suppression of a range of pro-apoptotic proteins through phosphorylation.

(b) **True.** Akt depends on binding to the second messenger PIP_3 for its function. PIP_3 is a phospholipid and is thus a component of the cell membrane. Attachment of Akt to PIP_3 anchors the protein to the cell membrane.

(c) **False.** The second messenger that activates Akt is PIP_3.

(d) **False.** Akt is a protein kinase.

(e) **True.** Akt directly promotes proliferation through phosphorylation and resultant inhibition of proteins that suppress cell growth at checkpoints, including p21, GSK3 and p27.

Answer 17: MCQ

See *Medical Biochemistry at a Glance*, 3rd edn (Water-soluble vitamins IV) or *Medical Sciences at a Glance* (Fat as a fuel).

(c) The transfer of fatty acids into mitochondria requires carnitine. Carnitine acyltransferase catalyses the reaction from acyl-CoA to acyl-carnitine, which then moves into the mitochondrial matrix in exchange for free carnitine. Here acyl-CoA and free carnitine are regenerated. Deficiency of the carnitine shuttle can be caused by carnitine acyltransferase deficiency and result in the presentation described.

Biotin (a) is required for carboxylation reactions. It is required for acetyl-CoA carboxylase and thus fatty acid synthesis in the cytosol. It is, however, not involved in degradation or transport of fatty acids. *Niacin* (b) or nicotinic acid is required for the co-factors NAD(H) and NADP(H). It is thus involved in most metabolic pathways, including fatty acid synthesis and degradation. However, it plays no role in the translocation of long chain fatty acids into mitochondria. *Adenosine* (d) is a nucleoside, not a micronutrient, that forms the basis for ATP and is a neurotransmitter. Although it forms the cell's energy 'currency' and plays a significant role in many reactions, it is not directly involved in the fatty acid transport into mitochondria. *Vitamin B_{12}* (e) is an important co-factor required for the degradation of odd chain fatty acids, specifically the final conversion of methylmalonyl-CoA to succinyl-CoA. It is not required for the translocation of fatty acids.

Answer 18: SAQ

See *Medical Biochemistry at a Glance*, 3rd edn (Glucose stimulated secretion of insulin).

Insulin formed in the body is derived by cleavage of pro-insulin in the Golgi complex (1). Cleavage yields insulin and C-peptide (2). Both are excreted into plasma where they can be detected (3). Synthetic insulin does not contain any C-peptide (4). Thus a patient who self-administered insulin will have high insulin levels but low C-peptide, whereas both will be elevated in the case of a tumour (5).

Answer 19: MCQ

See *Medical Biochemistry at a Glance*, 3rd edn (Acids, bases and hydrogen ions).

(a) Using the acid–base equation: $pK_a = pH - \log[\frac{[A^-]}{[AH]}]$, we know that $[A^-] = 1000 \times [AH]$. And since $[AH] + [A^-] = 6\,mmol/L$, $[AH] \approx 6\,\mu mol/L$.

Answer 20: EMQ

See *Medical Biochemistry at a Glance*, 3rd edn (Amino acids and the primary structure of proteins, Secondary structures of proteins and Tertiary and quaternary structure and collagen) or *Medical Sciences at a Glance* (Proteins).

(1) **D**. Secondary superstructures are short stereotyped 'motifs' formed from simple secondary structure elements.

(2) **G**. Co-operative binding of haemoglobin requires the ability of its subunits to increase the oxygen affinity of their neighbours after they have bound oxygen. Interactions between different protein subunits form the basis of quaternary structure.

(3) **F**. Ribonuclease undergoes post-translational processing that includes the addition of disulphide bonds. The disulphide bonds alter the protein's three-dimensional structure.

(4) **B**. α-Helices are a common simple structural element that is formed by regular arrangements of amino acids. This is the definition of secondary protein structure.

(5) **A**. The peptide bond is a covalent high-energy bond that requires considerable energy to be broken. All other interactions require less energy (heat) to be disturbed.

Answer 21: MCQ

See *Medical Genetics at a Glance*, 3rd edn (Autosomal recessive inheritance, principles and Allele frequency).

(e) From the description of this family, we know that all the couple's offspring will be heterozygous carriers of the CF gene. The probability that these children will pass on the CF gene is 50%. Assuming the population is in Hardy–Weinberg equilibrium, we now have to calculate the probability of them marrying someone who also carries a CF gene. The prevalence of the disease corresponds to freq(AA)=p^2, where p is the frequency of the CF gene in the population. Thus $p = \sqrt{\frac{1}{2500}} = \frac{1}{50}$. This is the probability of carrying the CF gene for each allele. The following table (Table 4.1) can now be drawn up. Thus there is a 1/100 chance of the grandchild having cystic fibrosis.

Table 4.1 Punnett square showing the probability of the family's second generation inheriting the CF gene.

	Second generation	
	CF gene	Wt gene
1/50 chance of CF gene	1/50 affected	Not affected
1/50 chance of CF gene	1/50 affected	Not affected

Answer 22: SAQ

See *Medical Biochemistry at a Glance*, 3rd edn (Absorption and disposal of dietary triacylglycerols and cholesterol by chylomicrons) or *Medical Sciences at a Glance* (Lower GI physiology).

Most fatty acids are initially emulsified by bile salts. This results in the formation of micelles and provides an increased surface area for the intestinal enzymes to act on (1). Emulsification is followed by degradation of triglycerides by pancreatic lipase (2), which removes the fatty acids at carbons 1 and 3, resulting in free fatty acids and 2-monoacylglycerol (3). The micelles then approach the brush barrier, where their contents are absorbed by diffusion across the membrane (4).

Short and medium chain fatty acids are digested in the mouth and stomach by acid-stable lingual and gastric lipases (5). They also do not require emulsification and micelle formation but can be absorbed directly (6).

Answer 23: MCQ

See *Medical Biochemistry at a Glance*, 3rd edn (Regulation of glycogen metabolism).

(d) Calcium stimulates several citric acid cycle enzymes as well as activating phosphorylase kinase via calmodulin. This results in glycogen breakdown and increased aerobic energy production that is needed for muscle contraction.

Answer 24: True/False

See *Medical Biochemistry at a Glance*, 3rd edn (Metabolism of carbohydrate to cholesterol, HDL metabolism and Absorption and disposal of dietary triacylglycerols and cholesterol).

(a) **False**. Bile salts are colourless, are mostly reabsorbed and do not colour the stool. The colour in the stool comes from bile pigments, especially bilirubin. Bilirubin is modified by gut bacteria to finally yield stercobilin, which gives the stool its brown colour.

(b) **False**. Bile is an alkaline solution that contains bile salts, pigments and cholesterol. It does not contain any enzymes. The emulsification of fat by bile and the subsequent creation of micelles do, however, enhance the action of pancreatic lipase.

(c) **True**. The liver synthesises bile salts. The gallbladder merely stores bile.

(d) **False**. Bile salts emulsify fats and aid the formation of micelles. Chylomicrons are fatty droplets formed by enterocytes and secreted into the lymphatics, but are not found in the gut. They also do not contain bile constituents.

(e) **False**. Bilirubin is a waste product from the breakdown of haem, and the liver exerts no control over its production. The liver will continue conjugating bilirubin, but as it can no longer be excreted via the gut, it will accumulate in the bloodstream and urine, causing jaundice and dark urine.

Answer 25: MCQ

See *Medical Biochemistry at a Glance*, 3rd edn (Transcription of DNA to make messenger RNA).

(c) snRNPs are small RNA–protein complexes that play an important role in splicing. Splicing is an important part of post-transcriptional modification.

Answer 26: True/False

See *Medical Biochemistry at a Glance*, 3rd edn (Fate of glucose in liver and Metabolism of carbohydrate to cholesterol).

G6PD is an important enzyme in the pentose phosphate pathway (PPP, hexose monophosphate shunt). It catalyses the irreversible reaction from glucose-6-phosphate to 6-phosphogluconolactone. The pentose phosphate pathway results in the formation of 2 NADPH from 2 NADP.

(a) **False**. The PPP is not required for amino acid biosynthesis. Amino acids are synthesised from intermediates of glycolysis and the citric acid cycle.

(b) **True**. NADPH is required for fatty acid biosynthesis and the pathway is thus highly active in liver cells, adipocytes and mammary cells.

(c) **False**. Oxidative phosphorylation requires NADH, not NADPH.

(d) **True**. NADPH is an important co-factor required for the reduction of glutathione. The reduced form of glutathione is important in the chemical detoxification of hydrogen peroxide, a reactive oxygen species. The inability to deal with toxins causes the haemolysis seen in G6PD deficiency. Red cells are affected, as other tissues have other enzymes in the citric acid cycle that can produce NADPH and reduce glutathione.

(e) **True**. The PPP provides the pentose sugars needed for the backbone of DNA and RNA.

Answer 27: EMQ

See *Medical Biochemistry at a Glance*, 3rd edn (**Enzymes: nomenclature, kinetics and inhibitors**).

(1) **C**. An increase in K_m is seen with competitive inhibition. Methotrexate competes with dihydrofolate for the active site of dihydrofolate reductase. It does this successfully, as its affinity for dihydrofolate reductase is one thousandfold larger than that of folate.

(2) **F**. ATP is both a substrate and an allosteric inhibitor of PFK-1. Therefore it is a homotropic effector.

(3) **G**. Citrate is not a substrate for PFK-1, but is an allosteric inhibitor of the enzyme. It is thus called heterotropic.

(4) **C**. The X intercept is equal to $-\frac{1}{K_m}$. A right-shift of the X intercept is thus equivalent to an increase of K_m which is seen in the presence of a competitive inhibitor.

(5) **E**. Aspirin covalently binds to cyclo-oxygenase and irreversibly inhibits the enzyme, which is reflected in a decreased V_{max} which persists.

Answer 28: MCQ

See *Medical Genetics at a Glance*, 3rd edn (**Mendel's laws**).

(e) This question assesses the basic terminology of Mendelian inheritance. Blood group A is the blood's *phenotype* in this case (e). The *character* (d) is the category in question, i.e. the blood group. A *gene* (b) is a unit of inheritance, which can be located within the genome: in our case the blood group gene. An *allele* (c) is any possible DNA sequence at this site, in this case the three known alleles I^A, I^B or I^O (this is simplified – actually there are hundreds of different alleles that can be subdivided into the three groups). Finally, the *genotype* (d) is the particular genetic make-up of that individual with regard to the gene; in our case the patient will be AA or AO.

Answer 29: SAQ

See *Medical Biochemistry at a Glance*, 3rd edn (**Genetic imprinting and Dynamic mutation**).

Trinucleotide repeats (usually CNG, where N is any base pair) can occur as these sequences are able to form secondary structures such as hairpin-like structures (1), which may result in shifting of the reading frame during mitosis, or during the repair process of DNA breaks and resultant expansion of the repeat structure (2). However, other multi-nucleotide repeats are not uncommon, and dinucleotide repeats may be both more unstable and more frequent than trinucleotide repeats, especially within satellite sequences (3). However, the human genome is based on trinucleotide codons which encode proteins (4), and thus trinucleotide repeats have the advantage of not shifting the reading frame and not running the risk of introducing nonsense mutations (5).

Answer 30: MCQ

See *Medical Biochemistry at a Glance*, 3rd edn (**Alcohol metabolism**).

(c) The metabolism of alcohol in the liver results in a high $NADH:NAD^+$ ratio in the liver. This inhibits gluconeogenesis as it causes malate dehydrogenase to reduce oxaloacetate to malate. It also results in stimulation of lactic acid production, giving a hyperlactataemia (d). Although alcohol inhibits the Krebs cycle it does not affect the respiratory chain (e). Insulin and glucagon do not play a direct role in alcohol-induced hypoglycaemia.

5 Physiology exam 1

Questions

Question 1: MCQ

As you read this question your eyes are stimulated to recognise the different colours surrounding your visual fields. Which *one* of the following statements is true?

(a) Cones can have pigments sensitive to one of three different colours: blue, green or yellow.
(b) Rods and cones show increased sensitivity to light upon prolonged exposure to bright light.
(c) The amacrine cells of the retina transmit signals from the eye into the central nervous system.
(d) Ganglion cells transmit continuous impulses even in the absence of stimulation.
(e) Horizontal cells are stimulatory cells that amplify the signals from the rods and cones.

Question 2: EMQ

A Erythropoietin
B Endothelin
C Nitric oxide
D Acetylcholine
E Noradrenaline
F Dihydropyridine
G Angiotensin II
H Atrial natriuretic peptide
I   B-type natriuretic peptide
J   Prostacyclin (PGI$_2$)

For each of the scenarios below, choose the most appropriate answer from the list above.

(1) Deficient in chronic renal failure and responds to counteract a decrease in oxygen transport to the tissues.
(2) Vasodilation secondary to shear stress occurs due to release of …
(3) Released in response to cardiac ventricular stretch and used as a marker of cardiac failure.
(4) Release stimulates miosis, salivation and sweating.
(5) Produced by the endothelium, causing vasodilation and inhibiting platelet aggregation.

Question 3: MCQ

A 7-year-old boy slips while walking, which causes a sudden muscle stretch resulting in a contraction. Which *one* of the following is true regarding the muscle stretch reflex?

(a) Golgi organs on the muscle belly discharge continuous information regarding muscle length.
(b) Intrafusal muscle fibres contract in response to stimulation by type Aα motor neurons.
(c) Group Ia and II afferent fibres innervate the muscle spindle.
(d) Primary afferents transmit information from nuclear bag intrafusal fibres only.
(e) The sudden stretch is opposed by the static stretch flex lasting a fraction of a second whereas the dynamic stretch reflex maintains a prolonged response.

Question 4: MCQ

Our daily energy and nutrient requirements are possible due to the complex digestion and absorption of a wide variety of compounds. What is the mechanism of glucose absorption?

(a) Apical membrane GLUT allowing facilitated diffusion.
(b) Through the formation of chylomicrons that are released into the circulation.
(c) Secondary active transport with Na$^+$.
(d) Primary active transport by glucose ATPase.
(e) Secondary active transport using gradient created by H$^+$-K$^+$ ATPase.

Question 5: SAQ (5 points)

Describe the sequence of steps after action potential generation in the skeletal muscle that leads to the muscle contraction allowing you to write the answer to this question.

Question 6: True/False

The function of enzyme systems in the body is influenced by the proton concentration, i.e. pH. Which of the following are true regarding regulation of acid–base balance?

(a) The normal arterial blood pH ranges from 7.35 to 7.45.
(b) The most important buffer system in extracellular fluid is represented by:
$$CO_2 + H_2O \leftrightarrow H_2CO_3 \leftrightarrow H^+ + HCO_3^-.$$
(c) The phosphate buffer system is an important extracellular buffer.
(d) Opioid toxicity results in hypoventilation, causing a decrease in O$_2$ partial pressure and decreasing HCO$_3^-$ production to cause acidosis.
(e) The respiratory response to deviations in blood pH is regulated by central and peripheral chemoreceptors, the latter located in the carotid artery and aorta.

Question 7: MCQ

A blind woman travels by bus. She is standing up. As the bus accelerates she notices this and is able to counter-balance by holding one of the rails. Which *one* of the following is true regarding this response?

(a) The acceleration causes relative endolymph flow in the semicircular canals which is signalled by hair cells.
(b) Bending of the ampullary cupula in one direction bends the cilia embedded in it, resulting in an increase in discharge.
(c) Otoliths' greater inertia relative to the fluid causes deviation of stereocilia of the hair cells.
(d) Crista ampullaris deviates posteriorly with hair cell excitation in the anterior ducts.
(e) None of the above.

Question 8: EMQ

A 33
B 40
C 100

D 8
E 150
F 3
G 122
H 55
I 6

For each scenario below, choose the most likely answer from the list above.
(1) A 35 year old with a 2-day history of vomiting has a bicarbonate of … mEq/L.
(2) A fit and well medical student's pO_2 on arterial blood gas in mmHg.
(3) Serum sodium concentration (in mEq/L) in a 56 year old with cerebral malignancy suffering from syndrome of inappropriate antidiuretic hormone (SIADH).
(4) Serum potassium concentration in a 42 year old with an arterial pH of 7.25.
(5) Serum corrected calcium (in mmol/L) in a 42 year old with parathyroid gland hyperplasia.

Question 9: MCQ

Sensory information such as visual, auditory and proprioceptive input is vital for adapting to second-to-second changes in our environment. Which of the following structures act as a major relay for ascending sensory information before projecting to the cerebral cortex?
(a) Substantia nigra
(b) Thalamus
(c) Amygdala
(d) Caudate
(e) Hippocampus

Question 10: MCQ

A 42-year-old man presents with dyspepsia secondary to peptic ulcer formation. Which of the following is true regarding gastric secretion?
(a) Gastric acid secretion is stimulated by enterochromaffin-like secretion of histamine.
(b) The H^+-K^+ATPase on parietal cells secretes protons into the lumen in exchange for K^+.
(c) Na^+ is actively transported out of and Cl^- into the lumen of the canaliculus.
(d) Carbonic anhydrase catalyses the production of protons.
(e) Surface mucous cells secrete an alkaline viscous mucous lining to protect the gastric wall.
(f) All of the above.

Question 11: True/False

During abdominal surgery, the surgeon notices rhythmic contraction of the small intestine and manipulation seems to affect the intestinal motility. Which of the following is true regarding gastrointestinal motility?
(a) There is continual intrinsic electrical activity along the muscle fibres that is modulated by stretch and the autonomic nervous system.
(b) The smooth muscle produces spike potentials as the cells depolarise during a slow wave, mediated through entry of calcium and sodium channels.

(c) Stimulation from the mesenteric ganglia increases gastrointestinal motility and blood flow.
(d) The enteric nervous system lies within the gut wall consisting of the Auerbach's and Meissner's plexuses which control smooth muscle activity, and local secretion and absorption.
(e) Cholecystokinin secreted by jejunal and duodenal mucosa inhibits gallbladder and gastric motility.

Question 12: MCQ

As a medical student climbs a mountain, the environmental temperature drops but her body responds to prevent core body temperature from dropping in order to maintain normal function. Which *one* of the following helps maintain core temperature in this situation?
(a) Feedback from temperature sensors in the brainstem to the subthalamic nucleus, which regulates homeostatic mechanisms.
(b) Parasympathetic stimulation to cause piloerection to entrap an insulating layer of air to reduce heat loss.
(c) The posterior hypothalamus sympathetic centres are stimulated to cause vasoconstriction at the skin.
(d) Hypothalamic mechanisms reduce heat production to reduce heat and energy loss.
(e) Sympathetic nervous system inhibition prevents sweating at muscarinic receptors.

Question 13: EMQ

A Temporal summation
B Tetany
C Saltatory conduction
D Relative refractory
E Facilitation
F Long-term potentiation
G Accommodation
H Receptor potential
I Excitatory postsynaptic potential
J Inhibitory postsynaptic potential

For each description below, choose the most appropriate answer from the list above.
(1) A 34-year-old man presents with the demyelinating condition Guillain–Barré syndrome. He has weakness in the movement of his lower limbs due to impairment in …
(2) A 2 year old learns the letters of the alphabet due to synaptic plasticity. An enhancement of signal transmitted at synaptic connections between two neurons is one of the major mechanisms for plasticity and is called …
(3) A 63 year old post parathyroidectomy develops prolonged, involuntary muscle contraction due to high frequency of action potential stimulation.
(4) A greater than normal impulse is required to produce a second action potential.
(5) Response to switching focus of vision from distant object to nearby object.

Question 14: MCQ

A 12-year-old boy is brought in by his mother who is concerned about his poor growth. Laboratory testing by the physician finds a low growth hormone level. What is the reason for his short stature?

(a) A deficiency in growth hormone-releasing hormone secretion by the hypothalamus.

(b) Non-functioning pituitary adenoma.

(c) Increased somatostatin secretion by pituitary adenoma involving somatotrophic cells.

(d) Familial genetic predisposition to short stature.

(e) There is not enough information to determine the reason.

Question 15: True/False

A 100 meter sprinter injects testosterone to improve athletic performance. Which of the following is true regarding steroid hormones?

(a) Steroid hormones are lipophilic and thus have poor solubility, requiring transport proteins.

(b) Major effects are slow and produce longer lasting effects through modulation of transcription and protein synthesis.

(c) The adrenal gland primarily produces steroid hormones except adrenaline and aldosterone which have rapid actions.

(d) Cortisol and testosterone both act mainly through G-protein steroid receptors that increase intracellular cAMP.

(e) Although not a steroid hormone, thyroid hormones also act through nuclear receptors to modulate gene transcription.

Question 16: SAQ (5 points)

Activation of the cardiac β_1-adrenoreceptor has positive inotropic and chronotropic effects. What are the targets to produce these effects?

Question 17: MCQ

A 32-year-old recent immigrant from Nepal presents with general tiredness, hypersomnia, bradycardia, poor appetite, constipation and poor hair growth. On examination, the patient is lethargic and overweight. Which mechanism best explains the symptoms?

(a) Impairment in iodine attachment to tyrosyl residues.

(b) Increased expression of RANKL by osteoblasts.

(c) Reduction in pro-opiomelanocortin cleavage to release adrenocorticotropin hormone.

(d) Downregulation of renal 1α-hydroxylase.

(e) Ischaemia and necrosis of the left adrenal medulla.

Question 18: True/False

Which of the following is true regarding blood flow in the main compartments of the systemic vasculature, i.e. arteries, arterioles, capillaries and veins.

(a) The steepest drop in blood pressure is in the arterioles.

(b) Regional drop in pO_2 in the pulmonary circulation results in an increase in vasculature radii.

(c) The total cross-sectional area of the arteries is greater than that of the arterioles.

(d) Compared to subjects at low altitude, those acclimatised to the low pO_2 of high altitude will have higher flow.

(e) Constriction of an arteriolar bed would increase the net movement of fluid from the capillaries to the interstitium.

Question 19: MCQ

A 17 year old with type I diabetes mellitus injects short-acting insulin three times a day. Which *one* of the following changes does insulin produce?

(a) Increases GLUT4-dependent uptake of glucose in skeletal muscle and adipocytes.

(b) Inhibits glycogenesis and gluconeogenesis.

(c) Increases expression of GLUT1 in erythrocytes and brain.

(d) Stimulation of Na$^+$/glucose co-transporter uptake of glucose in peripheral tissues.

(e) Stimulation of proteolysis and lipolysis.

Question 20: SAQ (5 points)

Upon destruction of erythrocytes, haemoglobin is released. This is broken down to haem and globin. Globin is recycled. Describe haem metabolism and excretion.

Question 21: MCQ

Acetylcholine decreases heart rate through M_2 muscarinic receptors in the heart. The mechanism of the receptor is which of the following?

(a) Ligand-gated cation channel

(b) G-protein coupled receptor stimulating phospholipase C

(c) G-protein coupled receptor inhibiting adenylate cyclase

(d) G-protein coupled receptor stimulating adenylate cyclase

(e) Ligand-gated anion channel

Question 22: MCQ

The menstrual cycle develops the ovum and the uterus to allow reproduction. During the cycle, in which phase is progesterone highest?

(a) Luteal phase

(b) Menstrual phase

(c) Proliferative phase

(d) Ovulatory phase

(e) Fertilisation phase

Question 23: MCQ

Increase in thyroid hormones T_4 and T_3 has a wide variety of actions. Which *one* of the answers below best describes these actions?

(a) Increased sensitivity of β-adrenergic effects, e.g. positive inotropy

(b) Increase in Na$^+$/K$^+$ ATPase

(c) Development and growth of the central nervous system

(d) Increased glycolysis and gluconeogenesis

(e) All of the above are actions of thyroid hormones

Question 24: True/False

Guillain–Barré syndrome is a demyelinating disease of the peripheral nervous system. Which of the following is true regarding action potential conduction?

(a) The action potential travels at high speed but shows decrement in amplitude and shape after 100 cm.

(b) Propagation is only orthodromic due to sodium channel inactivation after an action potential.

(c) A smaller diameter axon has a higher internal resistance and therefore a slower velocity of conduction.

(d) Myelination insulates the axon, increases membrane resistance and decreases membrane capacitance.

(e) Aα nerve fibres are unmyelinated and demonstrate slow conduction in comparison to myelinated C-fibres conducting potentially lethal nociceptive sensation.

Question 25: MCQ

Of the several hundred million sperm deposited in the vagina, usually only one spermatozoon will fertilise the ovum. Which of the following occur during fertilisation?

(a) The cortical reaction helps the spermatozoon break through the zona pellucida.

(b) Fertilisation usually occurs in the uterus in preparation for implantation.

(c) The spermatozoon nucleus fuses with the polar body to form the male pronucleus.

(d) The corona radiata follicular cells are released after fertilisation to form the corpus luteum.

(e) The secondary oocyte completes meiosis II.

Question 26: SAQ (5 points)

Electrocardiography is the process by which we record the potential changes at the skin that result from the membrane potential changes (i.e. depolarisation and repolarisation) of cardiac muscle. Describe cardiac excitation as represented by the ECG.

Question 27: MCQ

During exercise, both the oxygen consumption and carbon dioxide production increase significantly. The physiological changes include an increase in oxygen diffusing capacity. What mechanism is involved?

(a) Migration of type I pneumocytes to reduce the diffusion distance

(b) Increase in haemoglobin concentration

(c) Increased blood flow through dormant capillaries

(d) Increase in minute ventilation

(e) Stimulation of medullary centres by significant decrease in pH

Question 28: EMQ

A Hippocampus

B Substantia nigra

C Broca's area

D Striatum

E Medulla oblongata

F Superior colliculus

G Inferior colliculus

H Wernicke's area

I Inferior olivary nucleus

J Cerebellum

For each of the descriptions below, choose the most appropriate area of the brain.

(1) Essential in forming the memory of the 21st birthday party, its synapses demonstrate long-term potentiation to achieve this.

(2) Receives visual input with topographical maps at each layer to help direct eye movements.

(3) Primary function of production of speech and close interaction with the temporal gyrus where language comprehension occurs.

(4) Controls voluntary movements through dopaminergic pathways to the caudate and putamen.

(5) Responds to afferent input from baroreceptors and chemoreceptors to orchestrate autonomic nervous system regulation of respiratory and cardiovascular physiology.

Question 29: EMQ

A Prolactin

B Growth hormone

C Thyroid hormone

D Thyrotropin releasing hormone

E Somatostatin

F Cortisol

G Oxytocin

H Placental lactogen

I Luteinising hormone

J Adrenaline

K Adrenocorticotropic hormone

For each of the scenarios below, choose the most appropriate hormone from the list above.

(1) Increased serum concentration in a 36-week pregnant woman which has led to the enlargement of the mammary glands and is inhibited by dopamine.

(2) Hypothalamic hormone acts at the pituitary and stimulates release of prolactin.

(3) Suckling by the infant results in stimulation of the hypothalamus to produce an endocrine response, allowing milk to be secreted by the nipple.

(4) Produced from pro-opiomelanocortin along with melanocyte stimulating hormone, to act on the zona fasciculata of the adrenal cortex.

(5) Decreases the release of growth hormone and thyroid stimulating hormone by its action on the anterior pituitary gland.

Question 30: SAQ (5 points)

Define the following volumes: tidal volume, inspiratory reserve volume, minute ventilation, functional residual capacity and vital capacity.

Answers to Exam 1

Answer 1: MCQ
See *Physiology at a Glance*, **3rd edn** **(Special senses: vision)**.
(d) Retinal ganglion cells have a basal rate of firing. This rate of firing can increase or decrease in response stimulation depending on the type of ganglion cell.

With the three different pigments (blue, green and red), cones allow us to detect all the different colours (a). In colour blindness, either green or red cones are missing. Cones contain a slightly different opsin component to their photochemicals than rhodopsin in rods. Prolonged exposure to bright light reduces the levels of light-sensitive pigments, thereby reducing sensitivity to light, known as light adaptation. The converse with an increase in photosensitive chemicals leads to dark adaptation. Changing pupillary size is another modality of adapting to variable light (b). In the retina, the cones and rods synapse with bipolar and horizontal cells which in turn synapse with ganglion and amacrine cells. Only the ganglion cells leave the eye (c). Horizontal cells are inhibitors and connect laterally between rods, cones and bipolar cells to provide lateral inhibition. The central area where the light hits is excited whereas the neighbouring areas are inhibited to provide strong visual contrast (c).

Answer 2: EMQ
See *Physiology at a Glance*, **3rd edn** or *Medical Sciences at a Glance*.
(1) **A.** Erythropoietin is primarily released by kidneys to increase erythrocyte production to improve O_2 transport to tissues, e.g. chronic pulmonary conditions, high altitudes.
(2) **C.** Nitric oxide, a vasodilator, is produced by the endothelial nitric oxide synthase in response to shear stress, acetylcholine and platelet factors.
(3) **I.** Released by the cardiomyocytes of the ventricle and promotes natriuresis and vasodilation. Similar action by atrial natriuretic peptide released as a result of atrial stretch.
(4) **D.** Acetylcholine released by the parasympathetic nervous system has widespread actions including on the heart, lungs, and GI tract.
(5) **J.** Functions through G-protein coupled receptors and works in balance with nitric oxide, endothelin and other vasoactive agents in healthy individuals to modulate vascular smooth muscle tone.

Answer 3: MCQ
See *Physiology at a Glance*, **3rd edn (Proprioception and reflexes)**.
(c) The muscles and tendons have two sensory receptors providing proprioceptive information: muscle spindles providing muscle length information and Golgi tendon organs located in the muscle tendons transmitting muscle tension information (a). Type Aα motor neurons innervate extrafusal fibres whereas γ motor neurons innervate the small, specialised skeletal muscle fibres known as intrafusal fibres (b). Group Ia (primary) and II (secondary) afferents innervate the muscle spindle. Both types innervate the nuclear bag intrafusal fibres but only the secondary afferents innervate the nuclear chain intrafusal fibres (d).

Answer 4: MCQ
See *Medical Sciences at a Glance* **(Lower GI physiology)** or *Physiology at a Glance*, **3rd edn (Small intestine)**.
(c) Glucose transporters (GLUT) allow facilitated diffusion and are involved in the transport of glucose in the *basolateral* membrane of intestinal epithelial cells (a) after glucose has been transported in through the apical membrane by a Na^+-glucose transporter. Fructose, however, is transported by GLUT in the apical membrane.

Answer 5: SAQ
See *Physiology at a Glance*, **3rd edn (Skeletal muscle and its contraction)**.
Activation of the voltage-dependent dihydropyridine receptors leads to Ca^{2+} release from the sarcoplasmic reticulum through the ryanodine receptors. The Ca^{2+} binds to troponin C, resulting in a conformational change of tropomyosin that uncovers the actin active site. The myosin head extends perpendicularly towards the actin active site by cleaving an ATP molecule and attaches to the active site. The head tilts, causing the filaments to slide, called the power stroke, and release the ADP and P_i. A new ATP molecule binds to the myosin head, allowing detachment.

Answer 6: True/False
See *Medical Sciences at a Glance* **(Acid–base physiology)** or *Physiology at a Glance*, **3rd edn (Control of acid–base status)**.
(a) **True.** The normal H^+ concentration is 40 nanoequivalents per litre (40 nEq/L). The pH is lower in venous blood and interstitial fluids due to higher levels of CO_2 released from tissues.
(b) **True.** The bicarbonate buffer system consists of a weak acid (H_2CO_3) and weak base (HCO_3^-). The kidneys and lungs regulate HCO_3^- concentration and CO_2 respectively, helping to maintain the function of the buffering system.
(c) **False.** The phosphate buffer system is not an important extracellular buffer. Phosphate is highly concentrated in renal tubules and in intracellular fluid, giving it a significant role.
(d) **False.** Although hypoventilation does cause acidosis, it is not due to hypoxia but due to increased pCO_2.
(e) **True.** The peripheral chemoreceptors are essential in responding to deviations in pH, pCO_2 and pO_2. The central chemoreceptors, located on the medullary surface, respond to changes in cerebrospinal fluid pH, typically a reflection of arterial pCO_2.

Answer 7: MCQ
See *Medical Sciences at a Glance* **(Sensory)** or *Physiology at a Glance*, **3rd edn (Special senses: hearing and balance)**.
(c) The vignette describes linear acceleration, which is detected by the utricle and the saccule. They contain maculae which have a gelatinous layer with small calcium carbonate crystals called otoliths. Stereocilia project into this layer. The semicircular canals respond to angular acceleration, i.e. rotation (a). The ampulla is an enlargement at one end of each semicircular canal with a gelatinous tissue called the cupula. The stereocilia of the hair

cells are embedded in the cupula (b). The crista ampullaris is the structure within the ampulla associated with the cupula (d).

Answer 8: EMQ

See *Medical Sciences at a Glance* or *Physiology at a Glance*, **3rd edn**.

(1) **A**. Vomiting causes loss of gastric hydrochloric acid, resulting in accumulation of bicarbonate.

(2) **C**. The oxygen partial pressure is 21% of atmospheric pressure and in the alveoli is ~105 mmHg. In arterial blood this is ~100 mmHg with pCO_2 of 40 mmHg.

(3) **G**. ADH increases renal retention of H_2O in the distal nephron without an increase in Na^+ absorption, causing a dilutional hyponatraemia.

(4) **I**. In metabolic acidosis, protons are buffered intracellularly and to maintain electrical neutrality, intracellular K^+ is shifted extracellularly.

(5) **F**. Parathyroid hormone increases serum calcium by increased bone, renal and gastrointestinal calcium absorption directly or indirectly through stimulating activation of cholecalciferol.

Answer 9: MCQ

See *Medical Sciences at a Glance* (Hypothalamus and thalamus) or *Physiology at a Glance*, **3rd edn (Introduction to the sensory system)**.

(b) With the exception of olfactory sensation, the other sensations are relayed through the thalamus; visual input reaches the lateral geniculate nucleus, auditory input the medial geniculate nucleus.

Answer 10: MCQ

See *Medical Sciences at a Glance* (Upper GI physiology) or *Physiology at a Glance*, **3rd edn (Oesophagus and stomach)**.

(f) Parietal cells secrete hydrochloric acid that reduces the pH to <3.5 and is essential for gastric protein function and digestion. Parietal cells also secrete intrinsic factor necessary for vitamin B_{12} absorption in the terminal ileum.

Answer 11: True/False

See *Medical Sciences at a Glance* (Upper GI physiology) or *Physiology at a Glance*, **3rd edn (The gut and metabolism)**.

(a) **True**. The smooth muscle of the gastrointestinal system has pacemakers that generate continuous activity without the need for central nervous system instructions.

(b) **True**. The slow waves are generated by the interstitial cells of Cajal, which act as pacemakers. As the cells depolarise, spike potentials, which are true action potentials, are generated. There is a slow entry of calcium and sodium ions that produce a longer action potential than seen in neurons.

(c) **False**. Postganglionic neurons from the mesenteric ganglia are sympathetic in origin, which inhibit the activity of the GI tract and oppose the stimulatory effect of the parasympathetic nerves.

(d) **True**. Also called the myenteric (Auerbach's) plexus and submucosal (Meissner's) plexus. The former lies between the longitudinal and circular muscle layers and the latter in the submucosa. The myenteric plexus is mainly concerned with regulating tonic and rhythmical contraction, and conduction of excitatory waves along the gut wall. The submucosal plexus controls the function of the inner wall, including secretion and absorption. Both plexuses receive innervation from the parasympathetic and sympathetic nervous system.

(e) **False**. Although cholecystokinin does inhibit gastric motility, it stimulates gallbladder motility (chole-cysto-kinin comes from the Greek for bile-bladder/sac-to move). It is released in response to lipids.

Answer 12: MCQ

See *Medical Sciences at a Glance* (Hypothalamus and thalamus) or *Physiology at a Glance*, **3rd edn (Hypothalamus and pituitary gland, Autonomic nervous system)**.

(c) The hypothalamus orchestrates core body temperature regulation and has its own thermal sensors detecting both drops and rises in temperature. Additional peripheral sensors are present. The hypothalamus stimulates sympathetic vasoconstriction in the skin and piloerection to reduce heat loss. It also stimulates heat production by shivering and increases basal metabolic rate and heat production. As core body temperature drops, the regulatory mechanisms are impaired. In freezing temperatures, the vascular smooth muscles are often unable to maintain tone and sudden vasodilation may occur. This can prevent frostbite by maintaining blood supply.

Answer 13: EMQ

See *Medical Sciences at a Glance* (Nervous conduction, Cell excitability) or *Physiology at a Glance*, **3rd edn (Conduction of action potentials, Biological electricity)**.

(1) **C**. Myelination increases the velocity of neuron conduction as it reduces ion leakage. There are breaks in the myelin called nodes of Ranvier with a high density of voltage-gated Na^+ channels. As a result the action potential 'jumps' from node to node in a process called saltatory conduction.

(2) **F**. Long-term potential is, as the name suggests, a persistent increase in strength of synaptic transmission resulting from increased stimulation of the synapse. This process is considered to be the major mechanism underlying synaptic plasticity allowing learning and memory.

(3) **B**. Without replacement therapy, complete parathyroidectomy will lead to hypocalcaemia associated with tetany secondary to changes in permeability to positive inward currents.

(4) **D**. After an action potential the voltage-gated Na^+ channels are inactivated, giving the absolute refractory period where a second action potential cannot be generated. However, as some of these channels recover (but while others are still inactivated), a larger stimulus can initiate an action potential during the relative refractory period.

(5) **E**. Accommodation is the process by which the refractory power of the lens of the eye is changed. This is achieved by changing the thickness of the lens by contraction and relaxation of the ciliary muscles.

Answer 14: MCQ

See *Medical Sciences at a Glance* (Hypothalamus & pituitary) or *Physiology at a Glance*, **3rd edn (Growth factors)**.

(e) Although the other answers are plausible, growth hormone is released in a pulsatile manner and therefore a random growth hormone level fails to add any useful information. The most common cause of growth delay is constitutional growth delay where the cause of a temporary delay is often idiopathic (unknown) or genetic (familial).

Answer 15: True/False

See *Physiology at a Glance*, 3rd edn (Endocrine control).

(a) **True**. Steroid hormones are typically synthesised from cholesterol and their lipophilic nature makes them poorly soluble in plasma and they circulate bound to binding globulins, e.g. sex hormone binding globulin for testosterone.

(b) **True**. Although there is recent evidence that most steroid hormones also have a set of rapid actions through cell membrane receptors, their major effects are considered to be through intracellular receptors that affect protein synthesis.

(c) **False**. All the hormones of the adrenal cortex are steroid hormones.

(d) **False**. As above – steroid receptors are typically intracellular receptors that act as transcription factors. Although the rapid actions of steroid hormones are still under intense study, there is currently no significant G-protein-coupled receptor identified for these hormones.

(e) **True**. Thyroid hormone receptors are nuclear receptors.

Answer 16: SAQ

See *Medical Sciences at a Glance* (Autonomic nervous system) or *Physiology at a Glance*, 3rd edn (The autonomic nervous system).

β_1-adrenoreceptor activation produces its positive chronotropic effect through two major mechanisms: (a) increasing the funny current (I_f) in the sinoatrial (SA) node to increase the rate of depolarisation; (b) increase in the voltage-gated calcium currents in the SA and atrioventricular (AV) nodes to also increase rate of depolarisation and speed of conduction through the AV node.

The positive inotropic effect is achieved by increasing the sarcolemmal voltage-gated Ca^{2+} current to increase Ca^{2+} influx and therefore intracellular Ca^{2+}. This also increases Ca^{2+}-induced Ca^{2+} release (CICR) via ryanodine receptors. Second, β_1-receptor stimulation leads to phosphorylation of phospholamban, a protein that inhibits the sarcoplasmic reticulum Ca^{2+}-ATPase (SERCA). Third, CICR sensitivity is increased.

Answer 17: MCQ

(a) The vignette describes the presentation of hypothyroidism which in this case is probably due to decreased iodine in the diet. Iodide is actively taken up by the thyroid gland and thyroperoxidase oxidises iodide and couples iodine to tyrosine residues on thyroglobulin molecules.

Answer 18: True/False

See *Medical Sciences at a Glance* (Cardiovascular physiology, Blood pressure) or *Physiology at a Glance*, 3rd edn (Blood vessels, Control of blood pressure and blood volume).

(a) **True**. According to Poiseuille's law, the change in pressure between two points depends on the radius to the fourth power, viscosity, and length. Although capillaries have the smallest diameters, the total resistance depends on the number of vessels, and there are more capillaries than arterioles.

(b) **False**. Unlike vascular beds in the systemic circulation, hypoxia in the pulmonary circulation causes vasoconstriction and therefore a reduction in blood flow according to Poiseuille's law. The blood is diverted to regions with improved ventilation.

(c) **False**. The total cross-sectional area is greatest in the capillaries followed by arterioles, small arteries, veins, arteries and aorta.

(d) **True**. Flow is inversely related to viscosity. At higher altitude the pO_2 is lower, resulting in increased erythropoietin to increase red cell mass and therefore viscosity.

(e) **False**. Constriction of the arterioles supplying the capillaries would reduce the capillary hydrostatic pressure, thus reducing net movement of fluid out of the capillaries.

Driving pressure = [hydrostatic pressure in the capillary – hydrostatic pressure in the interstitium] – [oncotic pressure in the capillary – oncotic pressure in the interstitium].

Answer 19: MCQ

See *Medical Sciences at a Glance* (Endocrine pancreas) or *Physiology at a Glance*, 3rd edn (Control of metabolic fuels).

(a) Insulin inhibits the use of other sources of energy usage and stimulates utilisation of glucose. It stimulates lipid (e) and glycogen synthesis and inhibits glucose synthesis (b). Erythrocytes depend on glucose for their energy supply and does not require insulin for uptake similar to the brain (c).

Answer 20: SAQ

See *Medical Sciences at a Glance* (Blood) or *Physiology at a Glance*, 3rd edn (Blood).

Haem is metabolised in the reticuloendothelial system into biliverdin which breaks down to unconjugated bilirubin, which is not water soluble. This binds to albumin and is transported to the liver. Here it undergoes conjugation with glucuronic acid, making it water soluble. This is excreted into bile. Bacteria convert this to urobilinogen. The majority is excreted in faeces as stercobilin but some urobilinogen is reabsorbed into the enterohepatic circulation and renally excreted.

Answer 21: MCQ

See *Medical Sciences at a Glance* (Cardiac physiology, Autonomic nervous system) or *Physiology at a Glance*, 3rd edn (The autonomic nervous system).

(c) The muscarinic receptors are all G-protein-coupled receptors. The M_2 receptor opposes the action of the β_1-adrenergic receptor which is a G-protein-coupled receptor (G_s) that stimulates adenylate cyclase to produce cAMP. cAMP then acts on protein kinase A which in turn phosphorylates various targets.

Answer 22: MCQ

See *Medical Sciences at a Glance* (Reproductive physiology) or *Physiology at a Glance*, 3rd edn (Endocrine control of reproduction).

(a) During the luteal (secretory) phase, the corpus luteum secretes progesterone to stimulate endometrial glandular development and secretions, preparing it for implantation. The placenta takes over the role to maintain pregnancy.

Answer 23: MCQ

See *Medical Sciences at a Glance* (Thyroid) or *Physiology at a Glance*, 3rd edn (Thyroid hormones and metabolic rate).

(e) Thyroid hormones produced by the thyroid gland have widespread effects on metabolism, cardiovascular function, childhood growth and development, sleep, respiration, etc.

Answer 24: True/False

See *Medical Sciences at a Glance* (Nervous conduction) or *Physiology at a Glance*, 3rd edn (Conduction of action potentials).

(a) **False**. The action potential is an all-or-nothing response at every location down the axon and therefore does not produce any decrement in amplitude or shape. It can travel at speeds of up to 120 m/sec depending on the characteristics of the nerve.

(b) **True**. Although local circuit currents from an active patch of membrane will spread both backwards (antidromic) and forwards (orthodromic), the action potential only propagates forwards due to the refractory period experienced by the region immediately behind the action potential.

(c) **True**. In a thicker axon the internal resistance is lower as there are more ions per unit length of the axon available to carry charge down the axon. Therefore the conduction velocity is correlated to the axon diameter.

(d) **True**. By increasing membrane resistance, myelination decreases ion leakage, allowing internal spread of charge to occur over longer distances. However, there are breaks in the myelin with a high density of voltage-gated Na^+ channels where the action potential can be generated. As membrane capacitance is reduced, less charge has to be added or subtracted to change the membrane potential.

(e) **False**. Aα nerve fibres are the fastest conducting neurons which are myelinated and have the thickest diameter. They transmit proprioceptive sensory and somatic motor signals. In comparison, C fibres are slow conducting thin, unmyelinated fibres.

Answer 25: MCQ

See *Medical Sciences at a Glance* (Reproductive physiology) or *Physiology at a Glance*, 3rd edn (Fertilisation, pregnancy and parturition).

(e) The secondary oocyte is halted in metaphase II and only completes meiosis II if fertilisation occurs. The spermatozoon head contains the acrosome containing enzymes which are released (in the acrosome reaction) to break down the zona pellucida. The cortical reaction occurs after one spermatozoon penetrates the zona pellucida, whereby cortical granules are released to make the zona pellucida impenetrable for further sperm.

Answer 26: SAQ

See *Medical Sciences at a Glance* (Cardiac physiology) or *Physiology at a Glance*, 3rd edn (Cardiac cycle).

Electrical activity originates in the SA node and conducted through the atrium, resulting in atrial depolarisation (represented by the P wave) (Figure 5.1). The impulse conducts through to the atrioventricular node which produces a delay to provide a margin of safety. The impulse conducts through the bundle of His and the Purkinje fibres to the ventricular myocardium; the PR interval represents onset of atrial depolarisation to onset of ventricular depolarisation. The QRS complex demonstrates ventricular depolarisation which is followed by ventricular repolarisation (seen as the T wave).

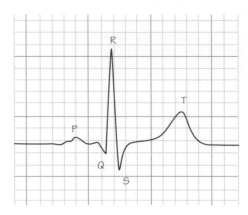

Figure 5.1 A normal ECG trace showing the cardiac cycle.

Answer 27: MCQ

See *Medical Sciences at a Glance* (Respiratory physiology) or *Physiology at a Glance*, 3rd edn (Ventilation-perfusion matching).

(c) During the resting state many pulmonary capillaries are collapsed while in others the blood flow is sluggish. The increase in flow through these vessels provides a larger surface area through which oxygen can diffuse.

Answer 28: EMQ

See *Medical Sciences at a Glance* (Structure of the CNS, Central nervous system function).

(1) **A**. Structures within the limbic system are important in the formation of memories. The hippocampus is vital for the formation of autobiographical and spatial memory. For example, damage to the hippocampus may lead to non-recognition of a person's wife but he may still learn how to play the guitar. There is still much to be learned regarding the workings of the hippocampus.

(2) **F**. The superior colliculus is involved in other spatial associated responses, e.g. head turns, attention shift.

(3) **C**. Broca's area is in the frontal lobe and damage is associated with expressive aphasia. Wernicke's area is located in the superior temporal gyrus and damage is associated with receptive aphasia.

(4) **B**. The substantia nigra consists of the pars reticulata and the pars compacta which contain GABAergic and dopaminergic neurons, respectively. In addition, it plays a role in eye movements and learned responses.

(5) **E**. The medulla oblongata receives afferent input from a wide variety of sources including gustatory input, proprioception and vibration sense, as well as visceral afferents. Therefore, it has a wide variety of efferent pathways making it critical in responding to acute change in cardiorespiratory physiology.

Answer 29: EMQ

See *Medical Sciences at a Glance* or *Physiology at a Glance*, 3rd edn (Endocrinology and reproduction).

(1) **A**. Prolactin levels increase as the pregnancy progresses to stimulate mammary gland enlargement and milk production. Suckling by the infant after birth continues prolactin and therefore milk production.

(2) **D**. The only hypothalamic hormone in the list is thyrotropin releasing hormone; oxytocin is also produced in the hypothalamus but released by the posterior pituitary. TRH stimulates release of thyroid stimulating hormone (TSH) but also prolactin release.

(3) **G**. Oxytocin is released by the posterior pituitary gland and its two major functions are uterine contraction during parturition and milk letdown during suckling.

(4) **K**. ACTH (adrenocorticotropic hormone) controls release of cortisol and is produced in response to corticotropin releasing hormone from the hypothalamus.

(5) **E**. Somatostatin is produced in the brain as well as by the δ cells of the islets of Langerhans and the small intestine. In general it has inhibitory actions.

Answer 30: SAQ

See *Medical Sciences at a Glance* **(Respiratory physiology) or** *Physiology at a Glance*, **3rd edn (Lung mechanics)**.

Tidal volume: volume of air inspired or expired with each normal breath (1).

Inspiratory reserve volume: the maximum volume of air that can be inspired after normal tidal volume (expiratory reserve volume = maximum volume of air that can be expired forcefully after normal tidal expiration) (2).

Minute ventilation: volume of air inspired or expired by a person's lungs in a minute, i.e. product of tidal volume and respiratory rate (3).

Functional residual capacity: volume of air in the lungs after normal tidal expiration, i.e. sum of residual volume and expiratory reserve volume (4).

Vital capacity: maximum volume of air that can be expired after maximum inspiration, i.e. sum of inspiratory reserve volume, tidal volume and expiratory reserve volume (5).

NB: when considering pulmonary ventilation, 'capacities' are usually the sum of two or more volumes. Other definitions to note: total lung capacity = volume of lungs after maximum inspiration, i.e. sum of vital capacity and reserve volume; reserve volume = the volume of air that remains within the lungs after maximum expiration.

6 Physiology exam 2

Questions

Question 1: MCQ

Using the concentrations of ions in a hypothetical cell and the equation provided in Table 6.1, calculate the potential at which the net flux of K^+ inward and outward is equal.

$$E = \frac{60}{Z} \log_{10} \frac{[Y]_o}{[Y]_i}$$

$$Z = \text{valence of ion}$$

Table 6.1 Intracellular and extracellular concentrations of K^+, Na^+ and Cl^-.

Ion concentration (mmol/L)	Inside	Outside
K^+	150	5
Na^+	15	145
Cl^-	5	110

(a) −64 mV
(b) −69 mV
(c) −73 mV
(d) −83 mV
(e) −89 mV

Question 2: True/False

A 39-year-old alcoholic presents with chronic pancreatitis. Which of the following statements is true?
(a) The pancreas functions as an endocrine and exocrine gland.
(b) Insulin is secreted by β cells within the pancreas and increases serum glucose levels.
(c) The pancreatic digestive enzymes aid in digestion of carbohydrates, lipids and proteins.
(d) Pancreatic secretion is acidic as pancreatic enzymes require an acidic environment for activation.
(e) In Zollinger–Ellison syndrome excessive gastrin secretion from a pancreatic tumour can lead to peptic ulcer disease.

Question 3: MCQ

A patient with a long history of poorly controlled diabetes mellitus now has autonomic neuropathy and presents to his GP with a history of dizziness on standing up. What is the cause of this?
(a) There is an inner ear lesion resulting in vertigo.
(b) Anxiety and hyperventilation associated with previous falls.
(c) Impaired vasoconstrictor mechanisms.
(d) Poor chemoreceptor response to venous pooling.
(e) Hypoalbuminaemia secondary to proteinuria.

Question 4: EMQ

A Voltage-gated K^+ channels
B Voltage-gated Ca^{2+} channels
C Na^+/K^+ ATPase
D Voltage-gated Na^+ channels
E Hyperpolarisation-activated cyclic nucleotide-gated channel (I_f)
F Stretch-activated Ca^{2+} channels
G Plasmalemma Ca^{2+} ATPase
H Na^{2+}/Ca^{2+} exchanger

For each of the scenarios below, choose the most appropriate answer from the list above.
(1) In the sinoatrial node the channel that is activated at phase 3 of the action potential, has a reversal potential of −20 mV and is responsible for slow depolarisation in the pacemaker.
(2) Responsible for the rapid upstroke of sinoatrial node depolarisation.
(3) Activates slowly in an action potential to initiate repolarisation.
(4) Essential for the plateau phase of the ventricular action potential and providing release of Ca^{2+} from the sarcoplasmic reticulum.
(5) Inactivation of which channels reduce the rate of action potential.

Question 5: True/False

Which of the following statements is true (Figure 6.1)?

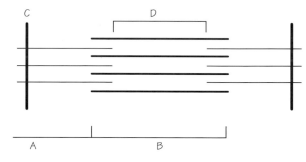

Figure 6.1 Schematic representation of a muscle sarcomere.

(a) The band represented by B contains myosin and actin filaments.
(b) The light band contains actin filaments represented by D and essentially involved in muscular contraction.
(c) The sarcomeric structure is preserved between the three major types of muscle: skeletal, cardiac and smooth.
(d) Titin is a large elastic protein that attaches to the Z-disc and thick filaments that produce the passive tension in muscle and aid in force transmission.
(e) The line represented by C is also called the Z-line (or Z-disc) where the actin filaments attach and lies between adjacent sarcomeres.

Question 6: EMQ

(a) Aldosterone
(b) Cortisol

(c) Vasopressin
(d) Adrenaline
(e) Parathyroid hormone
(f) Angiotensin II
(g) Glucagon
(h) Calcitriol
(i) Calcitonin
(j) Insulin
(k) None of the above

For each of the statements below, choose the hormone that best fits the description.
(1) A 72-year-old woman who is found on the floor dehydrated with a plasma osmolarity of 320 mOsm will release hormone to increase renal H_2O absorption directly.
(2) A 34-year-old man with hypertension, hypernatraemia, hypokalaemia and metabolic alkalosis due to an excess of …
(3) Stress hormone released by the adrenal gland has anti-inflammatory actions, causes gluconeogenesis and reduces bone formation.
(4) Severe hypomagnesemia will reduce release.
(5) Responds to hypoglycaemia by increasing gluconeogenesis and glycogenolysis upon release from the pancreas.

Question 7: MCQ
A 66-year-old man was found confused with suspected methanol poisoning. The arterial blood gas shows a pH of 7.25, HCO_3^- 16 and PaO_2 44 (on O_2). Which *one* of the following is likely to be a presenting sign?
(a) Widespread rash
(b) Increased respiratory rate
(c) Pupillary constriction
(d) Scratch marks
(e) Jaundice

Question 8: SAQ (5 points)
Discuss the steps occurring in the rod cell upon exposure to light, including inactivation.

Question 9: MCQ
The glomerular filtration rate (GFR) is determined by:
(a) afferent arteriolar pressures
(b) colloid osmotic pressures
(c) surface area of the glomerular capillaries
(d) glomerular permeability
(e) c and d
(f) a, b, c and d.

Question 10: True/False
A medical student wants to define ventilation and perfusion of the lung in an upright subject. He uses ^{133}Xenon either inspired or injected intravenously to evaluate these. Which of the following is true?
(a) Ventilation increases as you go up the lung.
(b) Perfusion decreases as you go down the lung.
(c) The V/Q increases as you go up the lung.
(d) In a hypoxic area of the lung, the perfusion increases.
(e) Impaired surfactant production would decrease V/Q ratios.

Question 11: MCQ
A 24-year-old woman is admitted with droopy eyelids and weakness that worsens as the day progresses. The physician diagnoses the patient with myasthenia gravis. What is the function of the most common target in this condition?
(a) Voltage-gated calcium channel
(b) Ligand-gated cation channel
(c) Breakdown of ATP
(d) Synthesis of aceylcholine
(e) G-protein-coupled receptor

Question 12: MCQ
During inspiration, intrathoracic pressure decreases, increasing cardiac preload. However, the Frank–Starling law of the heart helps maintain cardiac output. The law states:
(a) an increase in afterload results in a decrease in cardiac output
(b) cardiac contractility is adversely affected by increased inspiratory rate
(c) increased venous return results in increased cardiac contractility and stroke volume
(d) rapid cardiac response to challenges is maintained through tight sinoatrial node regulation
(e) fluid movement across capillary membranes depends on balance between hydrostatic and oncotic forces.

Question 13: EMQ
A Bifid P wave
B Small QRS complexes
C QT interval
D Tall QRS complexes
E Absent P waves
F Prolonged PR interval
G ST segment elevation
H ST segment depression
I P waves not related to QRS complex
J Peaked T waves

For each of the questions below, choose the correct part of the ECG change from the list above.
(1) A 66 year old presents with palpitations where the ECG shows unequal R-R intervals and a pulse rate of 140. Which ECG abnormality is common?
(2) A 52 year old with a history of hypertension and hypercholesterolaemia presents with severe central crushing chest pain. The A&E physician initiates thrombolysis treatment. What did she see on the ECG?
(3) A patient with acute renal failure is found to be hyperkalaemic (K^+ 6.3). What ECG change would be present?
(4) A 63-year-old man is found to have an ejection systolic murmur that radiates to the carotids on auscultation. The apex beat is heaving and the ventricular wall is thickened on echocardiography. What ECG change is most significant?
(5) First-degree atrioventricular block is defined by …

Question 14: MCQ
While climbing a mountain, a 37 year old experiences mountain sickness that could have been prevented by inhibition of carbonic anhydrase. What is the main effect of loss of function of this enzyme in the kidneys?

(a) Increased dissociation of carbon monoxide to shift the haemoglobin dissociation curve.

(b) Reduction in free radical production and therefore tissue damage.

(c) Reduction in urinary pH as a result of increased H^+.

(d) Increase in generation of new bicarbonate and excretion of excess H^+.

(e) Reduction in absorption of HCO_3^- and blood pH.

Question 15: MCQ

A medical student has isolated muscle fibres from the frog gastrocnemius and vascular smooth muscle. However, he becomes confused between the two. Which statement about the similarities and differences is correct?

(a) Smooth muscle requires <1/5 as much energy to sustain the same tension of contraction compared to skeletal muscle.

(b) Skeletal muscle depends on actin and myosin filaments for contraction, which cannot be found in smooth muscle.

(c) Healthy skeletal muscle and smooth muscle can demonstrate spontaneous electrical activity.

(d) Calcium binding to troponin is necessary to allow both smooth and skeletal muscle contraction.

(e) Smooth muscle demonstrates a fast onset of contraction and relaxation compared to skeletal muscle.

Question 16: SAQ (5 points)

Exercise challenges the cardiovascular system to provide the extra nutrient and oxygen supply required to meet the demands of the exercising tissue. What are the immediate and long-term changes the cardiovascular system undergoes with exercise?

Question 17: True/False

A 12-year-old South Asian girl demonstrates skeletal deformity including bowed femurs and a history of fractures. Which of the following is true regarding calcium regulation?

(a) The girl's symptoms may be explained by a deficiency of cholecalciferol due to poor sunlight exposure.

(b) Calcitriol acts at the intestine to increase calcium and decrease phosphate absorption.

(c) Parathyroid hormone increases production of calcitriol by stimulating liver 25-hydroxylase.

(d) Parathyroid hormone binds to receptors on osteoblasts to increase calcium and phosphate absorption.

(e) Calcitonin is another regulatory hormone that is released by the thyroid gland to reduce calcium levels.

Question 18: MCQ

After seeing a spider, a 22-year-old woman becomes tremulous, hyperventilates, feels tingling in her hands and eventually faints. What led to the cerebral hypoperfusion associated with this faint?

(a) Hyperventilation decreases carbon dioxide leading to cerebral vasoconstriction orchestrated by autoregulatory mechanisms.

(b) Fear caused a vagal response leading to bradycardia and cerebral hypoperfusion.

(c) Sympathetic stress response leading to widespread vasoconstriction including cerebral.

(d) Reduced cardiac output secondary to cardiac arrhythmias caused by adrenergic overstimulation.

(e) c and d.

Question 19: SAQ (5 points)

Spermatogenesis begins at puberty and continues throughout life under the stimulation of gonadotropins. Describe the steps that occur within the seminiferous tubules.

Question 20: MCQ

A 7 year old presents with a history of repeated epistaxis, prolonged bleeding on injury and bleeding gums. He is found to have an abnormality in glycoprotein IIb/IIIa function. Which *one* of the following is likely to be impaired?

(a) Activation of the intrinsic pathway of the coagulation pathway.

(b) Failure of calcium to interact with the platelet phospholipid surface for the coagulation cascade.

(c) Activation of plasminogen to plasmin.

(d) Platelet aggregation due to lack of fibrin interaction.

(e) Platelet binding to collagen exposed by endothelial damage.

Question 21: MCQ

A premature neonate demonstrates widespread collapse of alveoli due to high surface tension. What is the cause of this?

(a) Immature alveolar septum with lack of organised connective tissue.

(b) Lack of surfactant production by type II pneumocytes.

(c) Pulmonary hypoplasia due to diaphragmatic hernia.

(d) Interstitial fluid accumulation due to pulmonary hypertension.

(e) Neoplastic obstruction of the large airways.

Question 22: EMQ

A Distal convoluted tubule

B Proximal convoluted tubule

C Thick ascending loop of Henle

D Thin descending loop of Henle

E Thin ascending loop of Henle

F Collecting ducts and tubules

G Glomerulus

H B and F

I A and F

J None of the above

For each of the questions below, choose the most appropriate answer from the list above.

(1) A 65-year-old man who had recently started a statin presents with hyperkalaemia secondary to rhabdomyolysis. Which part(s) of the kidney will help to correct this electrolyte disturbance?

(2) In which part(s) does the Na^+-K^+2Cl^- co-transporter contribute to Na^+ reabsorption and help maintain the high renal medullary osmolarity?

(3) As a group is walking through the Sahara desert, they secrete large amounts of a hormone that inserts aquaporins into renal epithelial cells. Where does this hormone act?

(4) A 43-year-old emaciated man demonstrates impaired ability to concentrate urine due to reduced urea reabsorption. In which part(s) is urea absorption greatest?

(5) Laboratory studies in a 65-year-old woman with metastatic breast carcinoma demonstrate hypercalcaemia. Which part of the renal nephron responds by increasing calcium secretion?

Question 23: MCQ

Greater than 95% of oxygen is transported to the tissues by haemoglobin. The oxygen-haemoglobin dissociation curve can be displaced to the right by …
(a) Increase in pH
(b) Decrease in diphosphoglycerate (DPG)
(c) Increase in temperature
(d) Decrease in CO_2
(e) Fetal haemoglobin

Question 24: SAQ (5 points)

As you touch a hot stove, your hand is pulled away suddenly before you feel the pain. Describe the reflex activated.

Question 25: MCQ

During electrophysiology study of a neuron of the brain, an excitatory postsynaptic potential (EPSP) that has not reached the threshold for an action potential is recorded. Which *one* of the following is correct?
(a) An inhibitory signal arriving 5 msec after the EPSP would be ignored as the cell is in the refractory period.
(b) Stimulation by a GABAergic presynaptic neuron would increase the likelihood of an action potential.
(c) The postsynaptic neuron only responds to the largest stimulus when it receives input from multiple presynaptic cells.
(d) High frequency of impulses can lead to summation of impulses, increasing the likelihood of action potential generation.
(e) All of the above.

Question 26: True/False

A 43 year old is admitted following 24 h of haematemesis (vomiting blood). Which of the following is true regarding the homeostatic mechanisms that have been activated?
(a) The proximal convoluted tubule senses the reduction in renal glomerular filtration rate to initiate responses.
(b) Renin released in response stimulates conversion of angiotensin I to angiotensin II.
(c) Angiotensin II helps increase the glomerular filtration rate through efferent arteriolar constriction.
(d) Angiotensin II stimulates release of aldosterone by the zona glomerulosa of the adrenal cortex.
(e) Aldosterone acts at the collecting tubules and distal convoluted tubule of the kidneys to stimulate absorption of the K^+.

Question 27: MCQ

The compliance of the lungs is:
(a) roughly half of that of the lungs and thorax combined
(b) increased in pulmonary fibrosis
(c) decreased in pulmonary emphysema
(d) equal to the compliance of the chest wall
(e) roughly double that of the lungs and thorax combined.

Question 28: EMQ

A ATP
B Acetylcholine
C GABA
D Adrenaline
E Dopamine
F Noradrenaline
G Glutamate
H Nicotinic acid
I Muscurinic acid
J α-Adrenergic
K β-Adrenergic
L P2Y receptors

Fill in the blanks with the most appropriate answer from the list above.

The major neurotransmitter released by the preganglionic neurons of the sympathetic system is 1_____ and of the parasympathetic system is 2_____. In the sympathetic nervous system, the neurotransmitter acts on 3_____ receptors on postganglionic nerves. Postganglionic sympathetic nerves innervating sweat glands release neurotransmitters that act on 4 _____ receptors, whereas in the heart the target receptors are 5 _____.

Question 29: SAQ (5 points)

Digestion of a meal requires the integrated action of various types of cells within the gastrointestinal tract that are regulated through a variety of mechanisms including the GI hormones. Describe one major action and source of secretion (including cell type) for each hormone.

Hormone	Source (½ point)	Action (½ point)
Secretin		
Gastric inhibitor peptide (GIP)		
Motilin		
Somatostatin		
Gastrin		

Question 30: MCQ

The organ of Corti contains the sensory receptors for hearing. Which *one* of the following is true?
(a) Vibration of the basilar membrane depolarises medullary cells.
(b) G-protein-coupled receptors on hair cells release intracellular Ca^{2+} in response to sounds.
(c) Stereocilia on hair cells are bent as the basilar fibres bend.
(d) Movement of the oval window creates a wave along the tectorial membrane depending on the frequency.
(e) None of the above.

Answers to Exam 2

Answer 1: MCQ

See *Medical Sciences at a Glance* (Cell excitability) or *Physiology at a Glance*, 3rd edn (Biological electricity).

(e) The equation provided above is the Nernst equation used to calculate the equilibrium or reversal potential of an ion. For K^+ there is a concentration gradient (chemical force) driving the ion out of the cell but there is an electrical force driving the ion into the cell due to negativity of the membrane potential. The net flux depends on whichever of these gradients is larger. At the equilibrium potential the two gradients are equal and there is no net flux. The equilibrium potential of permeable ions helps determine the resting membrane potential of a cell. In this question +1 (valency of K^+ ions) is inserted for Z, 5 inserted for $[Y]_o$, and 150 for $[Y]_i$.

Answer 2: True/False

See *Physiology at a Glance*, 3rd edn (The exocrine pancreas, liver and gallbladder).

(a) **True**. The pancreas is composed of clusters of cells forming the islets of Langerhans which produce several hormones. Surrounding these clusters are the exocrine cells producing the enzymes necessary for digestion.

(b) **False**. Insulin is indeed secreted by the β cells in the islets of Langerhans and responds to increased serum glucose levels typically after digestion. It *reduces* serum glucose levels through increasing glucose uptake, decreasing gluconeogenesis and decreasing glycogenolysis.

(c) **True**. The pancreas secretes amylase (starch digestion); lipase, phospholipase A, colipase (lipid digestion); proteases e.g. trypsinogen, chymotrypsinogen (protein digestion).

(d) **False**. The pancreatic secretion contains bicarbonate to counteract the acidic gastric secretions entering the duodenum, and to modify the pH closer to the pKa of pancreatic enzymes. Secretin stimulates pancreatic bicarbonate secretion.

(e) **True**. This eponymous syndrome is associated with excessive secretion of gastrin, a hormone that increases gastric acid production leading to decreased gastric pH. Tumours are typically in the duodenum or the pancreas.

Answer 3: MCQ

See *Physiology at a Glance*, 3rd edn (The autonomic nervous system).
(c) One of the complications of DM is autonomic neuropathy. Upon standing, there is a decrease in venous return to the heart due to pooling of blood in the lower extremities (induced by gravity). This decrease in blood volume is detected by baroreceptors in the carotid and aortic arch that respond by stimulating sympathetic vasoconstrictor responses to prevent a drop in blood pressure. This patient has a failure in that response and therefore suffers from cerebral hypoperfusion on standing.

Answer 4: EMQ

See *Physiology at a Glance*, 3rd edn (The initiation of the heart beat and excitation-contraction coupling) or *Medical Sciences at a Glance* (Cardiac physiology).
(1) **E**. The HCN channel, also called the funny current (I_f) or pacemaker current, is a non-selective cation channel that along with the inward voltage-gated calcium current is responsible for the pacemaker potential in the sinoatrial node.

(2) **B**. In cardiomyocytes the calcium current (I_{Ca}) is carried through voltage-gated T-type and L-type calcium channels, the latter being more abundant than the former. The I_{Ca} is responsible for the rapid upstroke in the sinoatrial and atrioventricular nodes. This is in contrast to atrial and ventricular myocytes where the rapid upstroke is carried by voltage-gated Na^+ channels.

(3) **A**. Like neurons, the delayed activation of the voltage-gated K^+ channels is responsible for repolarisation of cardiomyocytes.

(4) **B**. The calcium influx through voltage-gated calcium channels is responsible for the plateau seen in the cardiac action potential and importantly results in calcium-induced calcium release from the sarcoplasmic reticulum, essential for cardiomyocyte contraction.

(5) **D**. The question discusses the refractory period (RP), which can be split into the effective and absolute RP. During the absolute RP, the sodium channels are inactivated and cannot trigger action potentials at all. As the membrane repolarises, some of the sodium channels are reactivated and an action potential can only be triggered by a stronger stimulus. This mechanism is similar to the RP in neurons.

Answer 5: True/False

See *Physiology at a Glance*, 3rd edn (The skeletal muscle and its contraction).
(a) **True**. B represents the A band containing the myosin filaments and where the myosin and actin filaments overlap.

(b) **False**. Although the light band does indeed contain actin filaments, it is represented by A and is called the I band. During myofibril contraction the I band shortens.

(c) **False**. Skeletal and cardiac muscle both have a sarcomeric structure. Although smooth muscle has actin and myosin filaments, they are not organised into sarcomeres.

(d) **True**. Titin also provides a structure for myofibril protein assembly. Mutations in titin can produce hypertrophic cardiomyopathy.

(e) **True**. A sarcomere is from one Z line to the next. The Z line is composed of filamentous proteins called connectins. Adjacent myobrils are attached at the Z line and therefore all the myofibrils are aligned, giving the muscle fibre a banded appearance.

Answer 6: EMQ

See *Physiology at a Glance* (Part 7 Endocrinology and reproduction) or *Medical Sciences at a Glance* (Hypothalamus & pituitary, Thyroid, Adrenals, Endocrine pancreas).
(1) **C**. Osmoreceptors, primarily in the hypothalamus and adjacent to the third ventricle, stimulate release of vasopressin (antidiuretic hormone) by the posterior pituitary. Vasopressin

stimulates increased renal H_2O absorption and causes vasoconstriction.

(2) **A**. Aldosterone is secreted by the adrenal cortex to regulate circulatory volume through increasing renal sodium reabsorption in exchange for H^+ and K^+.

(3) **B**. Both adrenaline and cortisol are stress hormones released by the adrenal (the former by the medulla and latter by the cortex). Adrenaline produces immediate second-to-second responses, whereas cortisol is a steroid hormone with a slower mode of action.

(4) **E**. Although mild hypomagnesaemia may increase release of PTH, significant hypomagnesaemia results in hypoparathyroidism and hypocalcaemia.

(5) **G**. Glucagon acts through G-protein-coupled receptors with primary actions in the liver and kidney.

Answer 7: MCQ

See *Medical Sciences at a Glance* (**Acid–base physiology**) **or** *Physiology at a Glance*, **3rd cdn (Control of acid base status)**.

(b) The arterial blood gas demonstrates a metabolic acidosis which is typical of methanol poisoning. The acidosis has a raised anion gap [Anion gap $= (Na^+ + K^+) - (Cl^- + HCO_3^-)$]. The compensatory mechanism for metabolic acidosis is hyperventilation to remove CO_2 and therefore raise pH. This is also the case in diabetic ketoacidosis, salicylate poisoning, uraemia and lactic acidosis.

Answer 8: SAQ

See *Physiology at a Glance*, **3rd edn (Special senses: vision)**.

Exposure of rods to light results in a conformational change in the photosensitive pigment rhodopsin to metarhodopsin II (1). This activates a G-protein, transducin (2), which in turn activates phosphodiesterases to break down cGMP (3). cGMP is bound to sodium channels, keeping them open (4). Thus, cGMP breakdown closes sodium channels, leading to cell hyperpolarisation, the receptor potential (5). Rhodopsin kinase, always present in rods, inactivates the rhodopsin to reverse the process (6).

Answer 9: MCQ

See *Medical Sciences at a Glance* (**Renal physiology: filtration and tubular function**) **or** *Physiology at a Glance*, **3rd edn (Renal filtration)**.

(f) Glomerular filtration rate is dependent on all the above factors. Movement of fluid out of the capillaries is dependent on the balance of hydrostatic and colloid osmotic forces across the capillary. The glomerular capillary hydrostatic pressure is determined by the pressure difference between the afferent and efferent arterioles. Normally the glomeruli are almost impermeable to proteins but this may change in disease processes. A reduction in glomerular capillaries, for example due to damage caused by diabetes mellitus, reduces GFR.

Answer 10: True/False

See *Medical Sciences at a Glance* (**Respiratory physiology, Respiratory pathophysiology**) **or** *Physiology at a Glance*, **3rd edn (Lung mechanics, Ventilation-perfusion matching and right to left shunts)**.

(a) **False**. The lung's weight causes the intrapleural pressure to be more negative at the apex than at the base. As a result, the lung base is relatively underinflated compared to the alveoli at the apex. Thus, the underinflated lung near the base has a greater compliance as it is on a steeper part of the pressure–volume curve. By definition, this produces a large volume change for the same change in intrapleural pressure.

(b) **False**. Similar to ventilation, perfusion decreases as you go *up* the lung. In the upper zones of the lung, the alveolar pressure far exceeds the pulmonary arteriolar and pulmonary venule pressures, causing collapse of the capillary and reducing flow. As you go down the lung, the pulmonary arteriolar and venule pressures increase, resulting in more positive transmural pressure that aids blood flow.

(c) **True**. Although ventilation and perfusion both decrease as you go up the lung, perfusion decreases more.

(d) **False**. In comparison to systemic circulation, in the pulmonary circulation blood vessels constrict in response to hypoxia to divert blood from poorly ventilated regions to better ventilated regions.

(e) **True**. Surfactant is produced by type II pneumocytes and reduces alveolar surface tension and therefore prevents collapse. Lack of surfactant would decrease ventilation as can occur in premature babies.

Answer 11: MCQ

See *Medical Sciences at a Glance* (**Neuromuscular transmission**) **or** *Physiology at a Glance*, **3rd edn (Neuromuscular junction and whole muscle contraction)**.

(b) Myasthenia gravis is an autoimmune condition affecting the nicotinic acetylcholine receptors at the neuromuscular junction. This is a ligand-gated cation channel that requires binding of two acetylcholine molecules to open. In another autoimmune condition, known as Eaton–Lambert syndrome, the target is the prejunctional voltage-gated calcium channels (a). Acetylcholine is synthesised by choline acetyltransferase.

Answer 12: MCQ

See *Medical Sciences at a Glance* (**Cardiac physiology**) **or** *Physiology at a Glance*, **3rd edn (Control of cardiac output and Starling's law of the heart)**.

(c) Otto Frank and Ernest Starling demonstrated this law through their studies on the frog and canine heart preparations, respectively. It underlies the heart's ability to respond to continuously changing cardiac end-diastolic volume (EDV). As the preload increases, the cardiac contractility increases to increase stroke volume, therefore keeping up with the preload. However, this works best up to a certain preload after which this effect is no longer seen. Do not confuse with Starling's forces that describe fluid movement across capillary membranes (e).

Answer 13: EMQ

See *Medical Sciences at a Glance* (**Cardiovascular pathophysiology**).

(1) **E**. Atrial fibrillation. In AF there is a random pattern of impulse generation from multiple foci in the atria giving a non-synchronised atrial myocyte contraction and thus absent P waves. These impulses are variably conducted through the AV node, which prevents all impulses from being conducted due to the inherent delay built in. It is the most common cardiac arrhythmia and causes stasis in the atria and increases risk of atrial thrombus formation which can produce cerebral emboli (i.e. stroke).

(2) **G**. ST segment elevation or new left bundle branch block represents severe ischaemia affecting the entire thickness of the myocardial wall, i.e. transmural infarct. It is preferably treated with primary percutaneous coronary intervention (PCI) or thrombolysis.

(3) **J**. Hyperkalaemia is a common complication of acute renal failure and can also be caused by several drugs, e.g. ACE inhibitors. K^+ determines resting membrane potential and therefore affects excitability of tissues. Typical ECG changes include tall T waves, prolonged QRS complex, flattened P wave and prolonged PR interval.

(4) **D**. The clinical examination suggests aortic stenosis with hypertrophy seen on echocardiography. Left ventricular hypertrophy is associated with tall QRS complexes.

(5) **F**. As the conduction through the AV node is impaired, the PR interval (represents onset of atrial depolarisation to onset of ventricular depolarisation) is prolonged. In complete (or third-degree) atrioventricular block, the P waves are not related to the QRS complexes (answer I) because the SA rhythm is not conducted to the ventricles and instead an accessory pacemaker lower down activates the ventricles.

Answer 14: MCQ

See *Medical Sciences at a Glance* **(Renal physiology: filtration and tubular function)** or *Physiology at a Glance*, **3rd edn (Control of acid–base status)**.

(e) Mountain climbing to higher altitudes causes hyperventilation due to the lower pO_2, leading to respiratory alkalosis (as CO_2 is blown off). This is compensated for by the kidneys by increasing HCO_3^- excretion that requires days. A carbonic anhydrase inhibitor, e.g. acetazolamide, pre-empts this by reducing HCO_3^- reabsorption by preventing:

$$CO_2 + H_2O \leftrightarrow H_2CO_3 \leftrightarrow H^+ + HCO_3^-.$$

Answer 15: MCQ

See *Physiology at a Glance*, **3rd edn (Cardiac and smooth muscle)**.

(a) Smooth muscle may use as little as 1/300 as much energy as skeletal muscle (a). This is essential as smooth muscle, e.g. in the bladder, often maintains a certain level of tonicity. Both smooth and skeletal muscle depend on actin on myosin for contraction (b). Smooth muscle does not contain troponin but instead calcium binds to calmodulin, which goes on to activate myosin light chain kinase. This is in contrast to calcium binding to troponin C to induce a conformational change in tropomyosin to uncover actin active sites in skeletal muscle (d). Healthy skeletal muscle is electrically silent, though it can display abnormal spontaneous activity when denervated (c).

Answer 16: SAQ

See *Medical Sciences at a Glance* or *Physiology at a Glance*, **3rd edn**.
Acute: intramuscular vasodilation to increase muscle blood flow (1), increase up to 25 times; and vasoconstriction in visceral organs to redistribute blood (2). The heart rate increases up to 3 times resting value (3). Along with the heart rate, the stroke volume increases to further increase cardiac output (4).

Long-term: myocardial hypertrophy (5) resulting in a larger stroke volume and therefore a slower resting heart rate. This allows a greater increase in heart rate during exercise (6). The ventricular size is normal or increased (7).

Answer 17: True/False

See *Physiology at a Glance*, **3rd edn (Control of plasma calcium)**.

(a) **True**. Vitamin D_3 (cholecalciferol) is formed by conversion from 7-dehydrocholesterol in the skin upon exposure to ultraviolet rays. Rickets may result from a deficiency caused by lack of exposure to UV rays due to excessive sunblock use, cultural/religious clothing and lack of sun in certain countries.

(b) **False**. Calcitriol (1,25-dihydroxycholecalciferol) increases intestinal calcium and phosphate absorption and decreases renal calcium and phosphate excretion. Parathyroid hormone increases phosphate excretion.

(c) **False**. Parathyroid hormone is essential to convert vitamin D to its most active form, calcitriol. The first step to forming calcitriol is to convert cholecalciferol by 25-hydroxylase in the liver to 25-hydroxycholecalciferol. The next step is conversion to 1,25 hydroxycholecalciferol by 1α-hydroxylase in the kidney, an enzyme closely regulated by PTH.

(d) **True**. Osteoclasts do not have PTH receptors and osteoblasts signal to osteoclasts by expression of RANKL.

(e) **True**. Calcitonin has a less significant effect on calcium concentration compared to PTH. It is released by the parafollicular C cells in the thyroid gland.

Answer 18: MCQ

See *Physiology at a Glance*, **3rd edn (Local control of blood flow and special circumstances)**.

(a) All tissues demonstrate autoregulation but the brain, heart and kidney (in that order) show the highest level of autoregulation. Cerebral blood flow is affected by metabolic changes, e.g. hypercapnia, hypoxia. Autoregulation also ensures that cerebral blood flow is relatively constant in the face of changes in systemic blood pressure usually between 50–150 mmHg.

Answer 19: SAQ

See *Medical Sciences at a Glance* **(Reproductive physiology)** or *Physiology at a Glance*, **3rd edn (Endocrine control of reproduction, Sexual differentiation and function)**.

Spermatogenesis occurs under the support of Sertoli cells stimulated by follicle stimulating hormone (1). The seminiferous tubules have a large population of diploid spermatogonia which continuously undergo mitosis to maintain supply and form primary spermatocytes (2). Primary spermatocytes begin meiosis and divide to form two haploid secondary spermatocytes (3). Each secondary spermatocyte enters meiosis II to form haploid spermatids (4). The spermatids develop a head and a tail, with the head composed of the nucleus and an enzyme-containing cap called the acrosome (5).

Answer 20: MCQ

See *Medical Sciences at a Glance* **(Blood)** or *Physiology at a Glance*, **3rd edn (Platelets and haemostasis)**.

(d) Platelet activation by ADP exposes gpIIb/IIIa on the platelet surface. gpIIb/IIIa acts as a receptor to bind fibrinogen required for platelet aggregation. It is impaired in Glanzmann's thrombasthenia and is also the target of several antiplatelet agents. Impairment in gpIa impairs binding to collagen (e).

Answer 21: MCQ

See *Physiology at a Glance*, 3rd edn (Lung mechanics) or *Medical Sciences at a Glance* (Respiratory physiology).
(b) Birth before 34 weeks is especially likely to cause respiratory distress syndrome due to lack of surfactant production which reduces surface tension. It is composed of mainly phospholipids and proteins. Glucocorticoid administration before birth can help stimulate surfactant production, thus preventing this potentially fatal condition.

Answer 22: EMQ

See *Medical Sciences at a Glance* (Renal physiology: filtration and tubular function, Renal physiology: loop of Henle) or *Physiology at a Glance*, 3rd edn (Reabsorption, secretion and the proximal tubule, The loop of Henle and the distal nephron).
(1) **F**. Plasma K^+ concentration is regulated carefully by the kidneys with the majority of the filtered K^+ being reabsorbed in the proximal convoluted tubule and the thick ascending loop of Henle. Secretion is performed in the distal nephron. A small amount is lost in faecal excretion.
(2) **C**. The majority of Na^+ absorption occurs in the proximal convoluted tubule and the thick ascending loop of Henle but this active transport mechanism also increases medullary osmolarity which provides the capability to produce concentrated urine and retain H_2O.
(3) **I**. The hormone described is antidiuretic hormone released in response to changes in plasma osmolality and to a lesser extent extracellular fluid volume. Aquaporins increase H_2O reabsorption and therefore concentrate the urine. ADH also has other actions including vasoconstriction.
(4) **H**. Urea is primarily absorbed in the proximal convoluted tubule and the medullary collecting ducts. The latter contributes to the high medullary interstitial fluid osmolarity.
(5) **J**. Calcium is filtered and reabsorbed in the kidneys but not secreted. Parathyroid hormone and calcitriol contribute to regulating the reabsorption.

Answer 23: MCQ

See *Medical Sciences at a Glance* (Gas transport) or *Physiology at a Glance*, 3rd edn (Carriage of oxygen and carbon dioxide by the blood).
(c) The oxygen–Hb dissociation is shifted to the right by an increase in H^+ (decrease in pH), CO_2, temperature and DPG. This phenomenon increases the release of O_2 at tissues.

Answer 24: SAQ

See *Medical Sciences at a Glance* (Sensory) or *Physiology at a Glance*, 3rd edn (Sensory receptors).
Nociceptive stimulus reaches the dorsal horn where it synapses with an interneuron in the interneuron pool (1). The interneurons synapse with each other and with anterior horn motor neurons (2). The motor neuron to the flexor muscles of the upper limb is stimulated (3) and antagonist muscles are inhibited (4). This is known as the flexor reflex (this response is elicited with any unknown stimulus). This is followed by the crossed extensor reflex whereby there is extension of the opposite limb to push away from the painful stimulus (5).

Answer 25: MCQ

See *Medical Sciences at a Glance* (Synaptic transmission) or *Physiology at a Glance*, 3rd edn (Conduction of action potentials).
(d) An inhibitor signal will generate an inhibitory postsynaptic potential (IPSP) and if arriving soon enough after an EPSP, there will be summation of the signals which may completely nullify the excitatory effect (a). Multiple EPSPs arriving from multiple presynaptic terminals can result in spatial summation and help reach threshold (c). Similarly, a high frequency of impulses can lead to temporal summation and an action potential if threshold is reached. GABA is an inhibitory signal which increases the net influx of negative charge and therefore will produce an IPSP (b).

Answer 26: True/False

See *Medical Sciences at a Glance* (Renal. Fluids) or *Physiology at a Glance*, 3rd edn (Regulation of plasma osmolality and fluid volume).
(a) **False**. A reduction in GFR results in reduced delivery of sodium (a marker for volume depletion) to the macula densa cells located in the distal tubule and associated with juxtaglomerular apparatus.
(b) **False**. Renin is released by the juxtaglomerular cells of the arterioles and functions as an enzyme to convert angiotensinogen to angiotensin I.
(c) **True**.
(d) **True**.
(e) **False**. Although the location is correct, the aldosterone stimulates Na^+ reabsorption (and hence H_2O) in exchange for K^+ and H^+. Angiotensin II is also able to directly increase sodium reabsorption by the kidneys in addition to aldosterone.

Answer 27: MCQ

See *Physiology at a Glance*, 3rd edn (Lung mechanics).
(a) The compliance of the lungs and thorax together is half that of the lungs on their own; in other words, the compliance of the lungs is double. Diseases such as pulmonary fibrosis decrease the compliance of the lungs. In pulmonary emphysema the compliance is improved, giving easier inspiration, but due to the loss of the elastic recoil, expiration is difficult.

Answer 28: EMQ

See *Medical Sciences at a Glance* (Autonomic nervous system) or *Physiology at a Glance*, 3rd edn (The autonomic nervous system).
Preganglionic neurons of both the sympathetic and parasympathetic nervous system release acetylcholine (**1 and 2 = B**), which acts

on nicotinic acetylcholine receptors (**3 = H**). Postganglionic sympathetic neurons use noradrenaline as their neurotransmitter in the majority of target organs, but in sweat glands they release acetylcholine that acts on muscarinic receptors (**4 = I**). In the heart the sympathetic nervous system releases noradrenaline, which acts on β_1-adrenergic receptors (**5 = K**).

Answer 29: SAQ

See *Physiology at a Glance*, 3rd edn (**Part 6 The gut and metabolism**) or *Medical Sciences at a Glance* (**Upper GI physiology, Lower GI physiology**).

Possible answers for the source and actions of each GI hormone are given in Table 6.2.

Answer 30: MCQ

See *Physiology at a Glance*, 3rd edn (**Special senses: hearing and balance**).

(c) Stereocilia are found on the apical membrane of the hair cells. As the basilar fibres bend, the stereocilia are bent, opening or closing the cation channels, leading to depolarisation or hyperpolarisation. Neighbouring stereocilia are attached by a thin filament.

Table 6.2 Gastrointestinal hormones, their sources and actions.

Hormone	Source (½ point)	Action (one for each hormone – ½)
Secretin	S cells of duodenum	↑pancreatic HCO_3^-, ↑bile acid secretion; ↓gastric acid secretion
GIP*	K cells of duodenum and jejenum	↑insulin secretion
Motilin	M cells of small intestine	↑migrating motor complexes†
Somatostatin	δ cells of pancreas; gastrointestinal mucosa	↓secretion of insulin and glucagon ↓gastric, gallbladder motility ↓pancreatic exocrine secretion ↓secretion of secretin, cholecystokinin, gastrin, motilin, VIP, GIP
Gastrin	G cells stomach antrum, duodenum, pancreas	↑gastric acid secretion ↑gastric pepsinogen secretion ↑gastric motility

*GIP is an incretin (along with glucagon-like peptide 1 – GLP 1) and is primarily stimulated by glucose in the duodenum. At supraphysiological levels it may inhibit gastric acid secretion but this function is primarily performed by secretin.
†Point can also be awarded for: 'increases intestinal and gastric motility/emptying'.

7 Pharmacology exam 1

Questions

Question 1: MCQ

A 46-year-old man is on phenytoin, warfarin, aspirin and glyceryl trinitrate (GTN) tablets. Which *one* of the following is correct regarding their metabolism?
(a) Phenytoin phase I metabolism involves conjugation with glucuronide.
(b) Phenytoin inhibits cytochrome P450 enzymes.
(c) Phenytoin undergoes oxidation to a polar metabolite.
(d) GTN swallowed has slow absorption but high oral bioavailability.
(e) Warfarin is a prodrug.

Question 2: MCQ

A 67-year-old type II diabetic on metformin and repaglinide presents with hypoglycaemia. What is the mechanism of the drug which most probably caused this side-effect?
(a) Decreases gluconeogenesis and increases glucose sensitivity.
(b) Inhibition of ATP-sensitive K+ channels.
(c) PPAR γ agonist.
(d) Mimics glucagon-like peptide 1 to increase insulin release.
(e) Dipeptidylpeptidase IV inhibition/

Question 3: EMQ

A Partial agonism
B Co-operativity
C Desensitisation
D Tachyphylaxis
E Competitive antagonism
F Chemical antagonism
G Physiological antagonism

For each of the scenarios below, choose the most appropriate answer from the list above.
(1) A 56-year-old woman on unfractionated heparin after a pulmonary embolism starts bleeding. Protamine sulphate is administered immediately. What is the mechanism of action of protamine sulphate?
(2) A 65-year-old man with benign prostatic hypertrophy is treated successfully with tamsulosin, which treats his hesitancy and restores a good stream. A few months later he is prescribed amitryptiline for restless legs syndrome and his urinary symptoms return. What is the interaction underlying the worsening symptoms?
(3) A postdoctoral fellow invents a new α-adrenergic agonist that has high affinity for the receptor. However, even at high concentrations the drug is unable to demonstrate the maximum response that phenylephrine can. What is the problem?
(4) A 46-year-old man is diagnosed with angina and started on atenolol. What is the mode of action of atenolol?
(5) A 76-year-old man with prostate cancer takes a GnRH analogue. How does it reduce the hormonal stimulation of the prostate?

Question 4: True/False

A junior doctor injects lidocaine into a cut before suturing a wound. Which of the following statements about lidocaine is true?
(a) Lidocaine will work better if there is infection or ischaemia around the wound as a lower pH environment results in increased efficacy of the drug.
(b) Lidocaine stabilises the inactivated state of the ligand-gated sodium channel.
(c) Lidocaine preferentially affects sensory fibres because it blocks sodium channels in a use-dependent fashion.
(d) Lidocaine has less cardiac toxicity than some other local anaesthetics because it dissociates readily from the blocked receptor ('fast in, fast out').
(e) 10 mL of 1% lidocaine contains 100 mmol of lidocaine.

Question 5: MCQ

A hypertensive man has recently started on lisinopril, an angiotensin converting enzyme inhibitor. He returns to his GP within days due to lip and facial swelling. What is the underlying mechanism?
(a) Decreased production of aldosterone
(b) Vasodilation caused by loss of angiotensin II
(c) Inhibition of bradykinin breakdown
(d) Decreased ADH production
(e) Increased cytokine release

Question 6: True/False

A 65-year-old man is evaluated by an ophthalmologist. On examination, pressures in the eye are high and a diagnosis of chronic glaucoma is made. Which of the following medication groups may be helpful in alleviating his problem?
(a) A selective β2-agonist
(b) A selective α2-agonist
(c) An acetylcholinesterase inhibitor
(d) A muscarinic antagonist
(e) A glucocorticoid

Question 7: MCQ

Treatment of myocardial infarction involves using multiple antiplatelet and anticoagulant agents to counteract the thrombosis occurring in the coronary blood vessel. One such agent inhibits ADP receptors. How does this decrease thrombosis?
(a) Blockage of glycoprotein IIb/IIIa activation
(b) Inhibition of thromboxane production
(c) Inhibition of phosphodiesterase
(d) Increased breakdown of fibrin
(e) Inhibition of glycoprotein IIb/IIIa

Question 8: SAQ (5 points)

A test subject receives a single intravenous dose of 1000 mg of a new medication with the test name ABC300. Table 7.1 gives the drug concentration at various time points.

Table 7.1 ABC300 plasma concentration in mg/L over a period of 10 h.

Time (h)	Plasma concentration (mg/L)
1	27.0
2	22.1
4	15.0
6	9.9
8	6.6
10	4.4

Given the information above, calculate the half-life, plasma clearance and volume of distribution, using the grid provided.

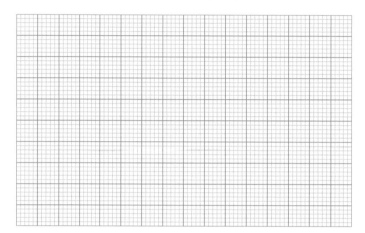

Question 9: MCQ

An elderly man is advised to take a daily aspirin following his myocardial infarction. Which *one* of the following is correct about aspirin?
(a) Enteric-coated tablets that prevent release into the stomach largely prevent the gastrointestinal side-effects of aspirin.
(b) The effect on prevention of cardiovascular disease correlates well with the dose.
(c) The cardiovascular effects of aspirin result from its selective inhibition of platelets.
(d) Aspirin is a competitive and irreversible inhibitor of cyclo-oxygenase 1 and 2.
(e) Unlike other NSAIDs, aspirin does not inhibit prostaglandin synthesis.

Question 10: SAQ (5 points)

Chemotherapy agents use a wide variety of targets to treat cancers. What are some mechanisms that are used to target cancer treatment?

Question 11: MCQ

The on-call doctor is called to see an agitated patient on the medical wards at 09:00 and she decides to prescribe intravenous midazolam, a drug with a plasma half-life of ~3 h. At what time would the plasma levels drop to 12.5% of the initial levels?
(a) 12:00
(b) 15:00
(c) 18:00
(d) 21:00
(e) 24:00

Question 12: MCQ

A 45-year-old patient with breast cancer undergoes chemotherapy. She has been feeling nauseous due to medullary activation and is given ondansetron. What is its mechanism of action?
(a) D_2 antagonist
(b) Phenothiazine
(c) Steroid
(d) Muscarinic antagonist
(e) 5-HT$_3$ antagonist

Question 13: True/False

A patient with newly diagnosed rheumatoid arthritis is started on methotrexate monotherapy. Which one of the following statements is true about this medication?
(a) Methotrexate is a competitive antagonist of dihydrofolate reductase.
(b) Methotrexate can be combined with sulfamethoxazole to achieve synergism.
(c) There is an increased risk of toxicity if trimethoprim is co-administered for a concurrent urinary tract infection.
(d) Methotrexate is conveniently taken only once a day when given orally.
(e) Methotrexate toxicity can be alleviated by the co-administration of folinic acid.

Question 14: EMQ

A CaEDTA
B Glucagon
C Glucose
D Naloxone
E Flumazenil
F Vitamin K
G NaHCO$_3$ (sodium bicarbonate)
H Oxygen
I Atropine
J No antidote

For each of the following scenarios, choose the most appropriate antidote from the list above.
(1) A 22 year old presents with headache, nausea, dizziness and confusion. She has been in a forest cabin for the past week with a wood fire. On examination, she has pink cheeks, is tachycardic and has normal oxygen saturation.
(2) A 56 year old who suffers from long-term depression decided to take an overdose of his antidepressants. He is admitted by paramedics after repeated seizures, which have stopped. His ECG shows prolonged QT interval and QRS complexes.
(3) A 63 year old has taken an overdose of lorazepam that he normally takes for anxiety. He is normally fit and well.
(4) A cardiovascular patient presents with tachypnoea, nausea, tinnitus and raised anion gap metabolic acidosis, after taking an aspirin overdose.
(5) A 21 year old is found on the street with multiple needle marks, slow respiratory rate and constricted pupils.

Question 15: MCQ

One of the major risk factors for cardiovascular disease is high cholesterol. This is reduced by statin therapy. What is the mechanism?

(a) Inhibition of gastrointestinal cholesterol uptake
(b) Decrease in lipoprotein lipase activity
(c) Inhibition of HMG CoA reductase
(d) Increased breakdown of cholesterol
(e) Decreased acetyl CoA synthesis

Question 16: MCQ

A woman develops chronic cardiac failure after many years of hypertensive heart disease. She is being treated with lisinopril, furosemide, digoxin and spironolactone. What is the mechanism of the drug that improves life expectancy?
(a) Inhibitor of Na^+/K^+-ATPase
(b) Diuretic acting on the Na^+/Cl^- co-transporter in the distal collecting tubule
(c) Diuretic acting on the $Na^+/K^+/2Cl^-$ transporter
(d) Angiotensin converting enzyme inhibitor
(e) Carbonic anhydrase inhibitor acting predominantly on the proximal tubule

Question 17: True/False

Basiliximab is a novel immunosuppressant monoclonal antibody that acts as an antagonist at the IL-2 binding site to prevent clonal proliferation of T cells. It is used to prevent graft rejection in organ transplantation. Which other commonly used immunosuppressant agents act on the same pathway?
(a) Azathioprine
(b) Cyclosporin
(c) Hydroxychloroquine
(d) Methotrexate
(e) Prednisone

Question 18: MCQ

A patient is admitted with severe renal colic and administered morphine intravenously. What is the predominant mode of action of morphine?
(a) Full agonist at the μ receptor, a G-protein-coupled receptor
(b) Partial agonist at the μ receptor, a ligand-gated ion channel
(c) Full agonist at the κ receptor, a G-protein-coupled receptor
(d) Partial agonist at the μ receptor, a G-protein-coupled receptor
(e) Partial agonist at the κ receptor, a ligand-gated ion channel

Question 19: EMQ

A Precursor uptake
B Synthesis of transmitter
C Uptake/transport of transmitter into vesicles
D Depolarisation
E Influx of Ca^{2+}
F Release of transmitter by exocytosis
G Interaction with postsynaptic receptor
H Interaction with presynaptic receptor
I α_2-Adrenergic agonist
J Inactivation of transmitter
K Reuptake of transmitter
L Breakdown of transmitter
M False neurotransmitter

For each of the scenarios below, choose the most appropriate answer from the list above.

(1) A 24-year-old woman sees the neurologist with spasmodic torticollis. An injection of botulinum toxin is arranged. What part of cholinergic transmission does botulinum toxin interfere with?
(2) A pregnant woman presents with a blood pressure that is persistently high with a reading of 164/94. She is started on methyldopa. What is the mechanism of action of methyldopa?
(3) A 54-year-old type II diabetic complains of depressive symptoms. She is started on a tricyclic antidepressant. How does this drug affect noradrenergic transport?
(4) A patient with newly diagnosed Parkinson disease is started on selegiline. What step of dopamine metabolism does selegiline affect?
(5) A patient with Parkinson disease is started on L-DOPA. A drug is added on to prevent peripheral side-effects of dopamine. What is the action of this drug?

Question 20: MCQ

A 7-year-old child receives a polio vaccine with a new adjuvant, which is a TLR-7 agonist. Which *one* of the statements below best describes how the adjuvant stimulates the immune system?
(a) TLR-7 agonists result in the activation of T-helper cells.
(b) Activation of the TLR receptor is an important step during antigen presentation.
(c) TLR-7 agonists stimulate macrophages and dendritic cells and serve to amplify the local immune response.
(d) TLR agonists increase vascular permeability.
(e) TLR agonists stimulate lymphocyte adhesion to the vessel wall.

Question 21: EMQ

A Arsenic
B Botulinum toxin
C Bungarotoxin
D Cholera toxin
E Curare
F Cyanide
G Nitric oxide
H Lead
I Malathion
J Pertussis toxin
K Saitoxin
L Tetrodotoxin (TTX)

For each of the scenarios below, choose the most appropriate answer from the list above.
(1) A patient receives a glyceryl trinitrate tablet to treat angina (chest pain secondary to coronary vascular stenosis). What is the active molecule?
(2) During an experiment, a scientist administers a toxin to prevent activation of voltage-gated sodium channels in the nerve axon, thereby preventing the upstroke of the action potential. What was the toxin used?
(3) A painter and decorator sees his GP because he is feeling unwell and slow. He is found to have a microcytic, hypochromic anaemia with basophilic stippling on blood film. Which of the above toxins inhibits haematopoiesis?

(4) A 5 year old is brought in by a distraught mother due to generalised floppiness. She reports that this happened soon after feeding the child canned vegetables. What toxin was probably involved?

(5) A researcher takes a toxin isolated from a deceased patient. He finds that when added to his cell culture, the G_s protein in these cells is continually activated through ribosylation by a toxin. Which of the above toxins has the described mechanism of action?

Question 22: MCQ

A 55 year old with hypertension, schizophrenia, gout and eczema presents 9 months after a change in his treatment. He complains of gynaecomastia and galactorrhoea. Which *one* of the following drugs may be causing this?

(a) Allopurinol
(b) Propranolol
(c) Topical betamethasone
(d) Haloperidol
(e) Cimetidine

Question 23: EMQ

A Lidocaine
B Flecainide
C Propranolol
D Sotalol
E Verapamil
F Amiodarone
G Procainamide
H Adenosine

For each of the scenarios below, choose the most appropriate answer from the list above.

(1) A 45-year-old patient presents with recurrent palpitations. He is found to have recurrent supraventricular tachycardias. After acute treatment he is started on an antiarrhythmic medication to prevent further episodes which proves highly effective. Unfortunately, 2 years later, he presents with progressive shortness of breath. A chest X-ray shows evidence of pulmonary fibrosis. What medication is likely to have resulted in this side-effect?

(2) A 21-year-old man presents with new-onset atrial fibrillation. He is given a Vaughan Williams class IC antiarrhythmic to convert him to sinus rhythm. Which of the above was used?

(3) A 22-year-old woman presents with palpitations. She has a regular heart rate of 190 with no P waves and is given an antiarrhythmic with a very short half-life. After administration, atrial but no ventricular activity can be seen on the monitor for 3 sec, after which she returns to sinus rhythm. Which of the above fits this picture?

(4) A 59-year-old asthmatic presents with palpitations. Her ECG shows fast atrial fibrillation. She is given an intravenous injection of a medication to slow her heart rate down without worsening her asthma. Which of the above drugs was most likely used?

(5) A 46-year-old woman with a recent diagnosis of Graves' disease (hyperthyroidism) describes palpitations and on examination is tachycardic with a bounding pulse. Which of the above drugs is most commonly used for symptomatic control?

Question 24: MCQ

A 49-year-old man with Parkinson disease arrives with visual symptoms and headache and is found to be severely hypertensive. He is taking selegiline and has just returned from a trip to France. You suspect a 'cheese effect'. How does the metabolite that builds up in the presence of selegeline exert its effects?

(a) It acts as a reuptake inhibitor.
(b) It stimulates postsynaptic adrenergic receptors.
(c) It stimulates presynaptic adrenergic receptors.
(d) It is an indirectly acting sympathomimetic.
(e) It inhibits the enzymatic breakdown of adrenaline and noradrenaline.

Question 25: SAQ (5 points)

A 75-year-old man goes to his warfarin clinic fornightly to check his INR. Give five conditions that are needed for drug monitoring to be worthwhile.

Question 26: True/False

A patient is admitted urgently with septic shock and is started on intravenous administration of noradrenaline as a vasopressor agent.

(a) The action is mediated through sarcoplasmic reticulum release of Ca^{2+} upon activation of phospholipase C in vascular smooth muscle.
(b) The effect is through activation of α_2-receptors found on vascular smooth muscle.
(c) The vasopressor effect is blocked by propranolol.
(d) The effect is mediated through a decrease in diameter of blood vessels.
(e) Intravenous antidiuretic hormone is an alternative agent that could have been used.

Question 27: SAQ (5 points)

For each of the rows below, explain the effect, if any, of the addition of medication 1 on the levels of medication 2 which the patient is already taking.

Medication 1	Medication 2	Effect of medication 1 on levels of medication 2
Ciprofloxacin	Warfarin	
Amiodarone	Digoxin	
Verapamil	Propranolol	
Isoniazid	Phenytoin	
Lisinopril	Rifampicin	

Question 28: MCQ

A 52-year-old man who presents with severe epigastric pain is found to have a duodenal ulcer on endoscopy. This ulcer is associated with chronic inflammation due to colonisation and often 1- or 2-week eradication therapy is undertaken. Which *one* of the following regimes is used?

(a) Clarithromycin, omeprazole, amoxicillin
(b) Omeprazole, ranitidine, bismuth
(c) Omeprazole, amoxicillin, ranitidine
(d) Clarithromycin, amoxicillin, metronidazole
(e) Lansoprazole, ranitidine, amoxicillin

Question 29: SAQ (5 points)

Chronic heart failure can result from the inability of the heart to maintain an adequate output to perfuse body tissues. Treatment is targeted to improve the physiological mechanisms impairing cardiac output. Discuss five treatments and the mechanisms involved.

Question 30: MCQ

A 45-year-old woman who has had a kidney transplant for polycystic kidney disease is taking regular mycophenolate mofetil to prevent graft rejection. What is the mechanism of its specificity for lymphocytes?

(a) Mycophenolate inhibits a pathway that has no alternative in lymphocytes.
(b) Mycophenolate targets rapidly dividing cells.
(c) Mycophenolate acts on a surface receptor only available in lymphocytes.
(d) Mycophenolate inhibits an enzyme present only in lymphocytes.
(e) Mycophenolate targets DNA found only in lymphocytes.

Answers to Exam 1

Answer 1: MCQ

See *Medical Pharmacology at a Glance*, **7th edn (Drug metabolism)**.
(c) The liver is the major organ involved in drug metabolism. This involves phase I reactions which cause biotransformation of the drug to a more polar metabolite, typically through oxidation (e.g. phenytoin), reduction (e.g. methadone) and hydrolysis (e.g. aspirin). Phase II reactions involve conjugation with endogenous compounds, e.g. glucuronide, acetyl and sulphate. GTN is administered sublingually as it is almost completely inactivated by hepatic metabolisation. Phenytoin induces cytochrome P450 enzymes.

Answer 2: MCQ

See *Medical Pharmacology at a Glance*, **7th edn (Antidiabetic agents)** and *Medical Sciences at a Glance* **(Endocrine pancreas)**.
(b) A common side-effect of repaglinide is hypoglycaemia. Repaglanide binds to a site at the ATP-sensitive K^+ channel. Metformin is less likely to cause hypoglycaemia and its mechanism is described by (a). Thiazolidinediones, e.g. pioglitazone, are PPAR-γ agonists (c). Incretin mimetics, e.g. exanetide, act through mechanism (d). Finally, DPP-IV inhibition reduces GLP-1 breakdown and includes sitagliptin (e).

Answer 3: EMQ

See *Medical Pharmacology at a Glance*, **7th edn (Drug–receptor interactions)**.
(1) **F.** Chemical antagonists, e.g. protamine sulphate, act by binding and inactivating the drug, which is heparin in this case.
(2) **G.** While tamsulosin is an α-adrenergic antagonist, amitryptiline has major anticholinergic properties and can worsen retention. Because the two medications act on two different receptors that result in opposing physiological responses, this is an example of physiological antagonism.
(3) **A.** This describes partial agonism. These agonists cannot produce the same maximum response as the *in vivo* agent, although the affinity for the receptor may be equivalent. This is related to intrinsic efficacy (the ability to demonstrate a response after receptor binding). A competitive antagonist has no intrinsic efficacy whereas a partial agonist has a reduced intrinsic efficacy.
(4) **E.** Atenolol is a competitive antagonist at the $β_1$ receptor, preventing agonists such as adrenaline and noradrenaline from acting on the receptor.
(5) **C.** Stimulation of the anterior pituitary by gonadotropin-releasing hormone as well as other hypothalamic peptides occurs in a pulsatile fashion. Continuous administration of a GnRH analogue results in desensitisation of the anterior pituitary and resultant decreased levels of LH and FSH.

Answer 4: True/False

See *Medical Pharmacology at a Glance*, **7th edn (Local anaesthetics)**.
(a) **False.** A lower pH does indeed increase the affinity of some local anaesthetics for the receptor; this includes lidocaine. However, before acting on the receptor, the local anaesthetic needs to penetrate the nerve sheath. Lidocaine has a pK_a of 7.9 and at physiological pH exists in both ionised (active) and unionised forms. At lower pH, the fraction of anaesthetic in the unionised form that can penetrate the membrane decreases and thus the drug is less efficacious at lower pH.
(b) **False.** Lidocaine does stabilise the inactive state (not the closed state) of the *voltage*-gated sodium channel.
(c) **True.** Sensory fibres, especially those of small diameter carrying pain, fire more frequently and have longer action potentials than myelinated motor fibres. Use dependence is an important explanation of the selectivity of local anaesthetics for sensory fibres.
(d) **True.** Fast-in, fast-out local anaesthetics such as lidocaine have less potential cardiotoxicity than fast-in, slow-out anaesthetics such as bupivacaine. Lidocaine generally dissociates itself from the channel prior to the next beat arriving.
(e) **False.** 10 mL of 1% lidocaine contain 100 milli*grams* of lidocaine. The molecular weight of lidocaine is 234 g/mol, thus 100 mmol would weigh 23 g. Even without knowing the molecular weight of lidocaine, it is easily deducible that 100 mmol of lidocaine will weigh more than 0.1 g (which is 1% of 10 mL).

Answer 5: MCQ

See *Medical Pharmacology at a Glance*, **7th edn (Drugs used in hypertension)**.
(c) Angiotensin converting enzyme (ACE) inhibitors not only inhibit the conversion of angiotensin I to angiotensin II but also inhibit breakdown of bradykinin. ACE inhibition does have many of the above effects (e.g. decreased aldosterone production, vasodilation) but bradykinin mediates the angio-oedema and cough sometimes seen in ACE inhibitor use. Using angiotensin receptor blockers (ARB) can avoid this side-effect.

Answer 6: True/False

See *Medical Pharmacology at a Glance*, **7th edn (Ocular pharmacology)**.
The principle behind the use of medications to prevent or treat glaucoma is to prevent the folding of the iris which happens during dilation of the pupils. Thus medications which favour constriction or prevent dilation of the pupil will be of benefit.
(a) **False.** Stimulation of adrenergic transmission in the eye results in dilation of the pupil and may worsen or cause obstruction of aqueous humour. Selective $β_2$-agonists have been reported to cause acute glaucoma.
(b) **True.** Unlike all other types of adrenergic receptors, $α_2$-agonists act on presynaptic receptors to reduce norepinephrine release, which results in a reduction in aqueous humour production.
(c) **True.** Cholinergic transmission causes contraction of the ciliary muscle and is enhanced by anticholinesterases. This results in tightening the trabecular meshwork which in turn increases aqueous outflow.
(d) **False.** Atropine was used in the past to cause mydriasis. It can worsen glaucoma.

(e) **False**. Glucocorticoids can rarely worsen glaucoma by decreasing absorption or increasing production of aqueous fluid. They have no place in the treatment of open-angle (chronic) glaucoma.

Answer 7: MCQ

See *Medical Pharmacology at a Glance*, 7th edn (**Drugs used to affect blood coagulation**).
(a) Thienopyridines, e.g. clopidogrel, inhibit ADP P_{2Y12} responsible for increased expression of activated GpIIb/IIIa that in turn binds fibrinogen, involved in cross-linking platelets. Aspirin inhibits cyclo-oxygenase-mediated production of thromboxane (b), while newer agents, e.g. abciximab, inhibit gpIIb/IIIa directly (e). Tissue plasminogen activator (tPA), e.g. streptokinase, promotes the production of plasmin essential in the breakdown of fibrin (d).

Answer 8: SAQ

See *Medical Pharmacology at a Glance*, 7th edn (**Drug absorption, distribution and excretion**).
To obtain a linear graph in a drug with first-order kinetics, it is first important to calculate the natural logarithms of the concentrations given above and plot them against time. This will give a y intercept of $3.5 = \ln(C_0)$. Therefore the initial concentration C_0 is 33 mg. The rate constant λ is the slope of the curve which is 0.20. Thus the half-life is $t_{1/2} = \frac{\ln(2)}{\lambda} = 3.4 \, h$. Given that $AUC = \frac{C_0}{\lambda}$, the clearance can be calculated as follows: $CL = \frac{D}{AUC} = \frac{D \times \lambda}{C_0} = 6.1 \, l/h$. Finally the volume of distribution can be calculated as follows: $VoD = \frac{CL}{\lambda} = 30.5 \, l$.

Answer 9: MCQ

See *Medical Pharmacology at a Glance*, 7th edn (**Drugs used to affect blood coagulation**).
(d) Aspirin is an atypical NSAID, which competitively but irreversibly inhibits both cyclo-oxygenase 1 and 2 (d), resulting in the inhibition of prostaglandin synthesis (e). It is no more selective for platelets than for other cells, but as platelets are not able to regenerate their dysfunctional cyclo-oxygenase enzymes, the inhibition is permanent in platelets (c). Given this mechanism, it is unsurprising that small doses achieve the same cardiovascular protective effect as larger ones and very large doses may in fact be counterproductive, as they would eliminate the useful antithrombotic effect of endothelial cyclo-oxygenase (b). Because aspirin easily reaches the stomach via the bloodstream, the mode of administration, whether rectal or enteric coated, has not been shown to alter the side-effect profile significantly (a).

Answer 10: SAQ

See *Medical Pharmacology at a Glance*, 7th edn (**Drugs used in cancer**) or *Medical Sciences at a Glance* (**Chemotherapy**).
Chemical modification of DNA, e.g. alkylating agents, platinum compounds
Interfere with synthesis of purines or pyrimidines, e.g. dihydrofolate reductase inhibitors, pyrimidine and purine analogues
Topoisomerase inhibitors
Inhibition of mitosis, e.g. vinca alkaloids
Cancer-specific targets, e.g. tyrosine kinase inhibitor used in chronic myeloid leukaemia, oestrogen receptor antagonists used in breast cancer

Answer 11: MCQ

See *Medical Pharmacology at a Glance*, 7th edn (**Drug absorption, distribution and excretion**).
(c) The plasma half-life of a drug is the time taken for the plasma concentration to drop by 50%. The body will continue to eliminate half of the blood concentration every half-life, i.e. for midazolam at time 0 h, the plasma levels are at 100%, at 3 h 50%, at 6 h 25%, at 9 h 12.5% and so on. Therefore the answer is 18:00 or 9 h.

Answer 12: MCQ

See *Medical Pharmacology at a Glance*, 7th edn (**Drugs used in nausea and vertigo (antiemetics)**).
(e) Vomiting is co-ordinated by the vomiting centre in the lateral reticular formation of the medulla and receives multiple afferents including from the chemoreceptor trigger zone in the area postrema. This area is not insulated by the blood–brain barrier and is therefore exposed to circulating agents (including drugs). The area postrema contains both dopamine (D_2) and serotonin ($5\text{-}HT_3$) receptors. Therefore, D_2 (e.g. metoclopramide, domperidone) and $5\text{-}HT_3$ (e.g. ondansetron) antagonists work well. It is not clear why steroids are antiemetics. Phenothiazines, e.g. prochlorperazine, have multiple effects but most importantly ae antidopaminergic. The vomiting centre itself has muscarinic and histamine receptors and antagonists at these targets also are effective antiemetics.

Answer 13: True/False

See *Medical Pharmacology at a Glance*, 7th edn (**Immunosuppressants and antirheumatoid drugs**) or *Medical Sciences at a Glance* (**Chemotherapy**).
(a) **True**.
(b) **False**. Sulfamethoxazole is an antibacterial agent that inhibits the synthesis of folate from para-aminobenzoic acid. It is not used in conjunction with methotrexate but is used to achieve synergism with trimethoprim. In the context of rheumatoid arthritis, sulfasalazine, another sulphonamide, has been used successfully in conjunction with methotrexate but as yet no definite synergistic (additive) benefit has been proven with this combination.
(c) **True**. Methotrexate and trimethoprim both inhibit dihydrofolate reductase. Although trimethoprim is highly specific for *bacterial* dihydrofolate reductase, it does also inhibit the human enzyme to a lesser extent and can thus augment the toxicity caused by methotrexate, which is also a dihydrofolate reductase inhibitor.
(d) **False**. Methotrexate dosing varies greatly based on the indication, and may be given daily in certain chemotherapy regiments. However, it is important to know that when used as an immunosuppressant in rheumatoid arthritis and inflammatory bowel disease, it is given *weekly*. Daily prescription of weekly methotrexate has in the past led to serious consequences.
(e) **True**. Folinic acid, a tetrahydrofolate analogue, replenishes the FH_4 stores that are depleted by methotrexate. It is usually given some time after methotrexate and can then 'rescue' gastrointestinal and bone marrow cells from methotrexate toxicity.

Answer 14: EMQ

See *Medical Pharmacology at a Glance*, 7th edn (Poisoning).

(1) **H**. The presentation is consistent with carbon monoxide poisoning. Carbon monoxide has more than 230 times the affinity for haemoglobin of oxygen and a pulse oximeter incorrectly detects normal oxygen saturation. The treatment is 100% oxygen therapy to hasten CO dissociation from haemoglobin.

(2) **G**. Tricyclic antidepressants are particularly toxic in overdose, making SSRIs preferable for depression treatment. In overdose, TCAs can cause cardiac arrhythmias, convulsions and coma. The first-line treatment is intravenous $NaHCO_3$, repeated as appropriate.

(3) **E**. Flumazenil is a competitive inhibitor of the benzodiazepine GABA receptor binding site. If a combination of drugs has been taken then flumazenil is usually avoided to avoid development of seizures that are difficult to treat.

(4) **G**. Sodium bicarbonate increases salicylate elimination by alkanisation of the urine.

(5) **D**. The signs are consistent with an opioid overdose which can be treated with the opioid antagonist naloxone. However, naloxone is a short-acting drug and repeated doses may be required.

Answer 15: MCQ

See *Medical Pharmacology at a Glance*, 7th edn (Lipid-lowering drugs) or *Medical Sciences at a Glance* (Cardiovascular pathophysiology).

(c) Hydroxyl-methylglutaryl coenzyme A reductase is the enzyme catalysing the rate-limiting step in cholesterol synthesis occurring in the liver. As a result of its inhibition, there is upregulation of LDL receptors in the hepatocytes and increased uptake of circulating LDL particles.

Answer 16: MCQ

See *Medical Pharmacology at a Glance*, 7th edn (Drugs used in heart failure) or *Medical Sciences at a Glance* (Cardiovascular pathophysiology).

(d) Drugs that are proven to increase life expectancy in congestive cardiac failure include ACE inhibitors, β-blockers and spironolactone. Spironolactone is an inhibitor of the intracellular aldosterone receptor. Other diuretics do not have a proven mortality benefit but are certainly needed for symptomatic control and are rightly ubiquitously used. Despite its widespread use, digoxin also has no mortality benefit (a). Carbonic anhydrase inhibitors have neither mortality benefit nor a role in the treatment of heart failure (e).

Answer 17: True/False

See *Medical Pharmacology at a Glance*, 7th edn (Drugs used in cancer, Immunosuppressants and antirheumatoid drugs).

(a) **False**. Azathioprine is a prodrug of mercaptopurine. Mercaptopurine acts as a purine analogue that inhibits purine synthesis.

(b) **True**. Cyclosporin is a calcineurin inhibitor. Calcineurin is responsible for activating the transcription of interleukin-2, resulting in decreased T cell function.

(c) **False**. The mechanism of the immunosuppressant action of the antimalarial hydroxychloroquine may be explained by its accumulation in lysosomes, resulting in alkalisation and thus in weakened phagocytosis and respiratory burst.

(d) **False**. Methotrexate acts to inhibit folate synthesis and thus is cytotoxic to rapidly dividing cells, thereby causing immunosuppression.

(e) **True**. Steroids are known to have a multitude of effects, including immune suppression. This is again mediated by multiple pathways, of which inhibition of interleukin-2 appears to be most important.

Answer 18: MCQ

See *Medical Pharmacology at a Glance*, 7th edn (Opioid analgesics).

(d) Morphine is a partial agonist at the μ receptor, which is surprising given its potency. Morphine is indeed capable of eliciting a very strong response, but it is submaximal compared with full agonists such as etorphine or methadone.

Answer 19: EMQ

See *Medical Pharmacology at a Glance*, 7th edn (Drugs used in hypertension, Drugs acting at the neuromuscular junction, Drugs used in affective disorders: antidepressants, Drugs used in Parkinson's disease).

(1) **F**. Botulinum toxin has protease activity. When it reaches the synaptic cytoplasm, it cleaves SNARE proteins that are required for synaptic vesicles to dock and fuse with the plasma membrane, and thus inhibits the exocytosis of transmitter vesicles.

(2) **I**. Methyldopa, like clonidine, is an α_2-adrenergic agonist which inhibits sympathetic output, thereby lowering blood pressure. Due to alternatives this drug is limited to use in pregnancy.

(3) **K**. Tricyclic antidepressants inhibit the reuptake of norepinephrine and serotonin, thereby enhancing neurotransmission. However, they are not commonly used due to their many side-effects and lethality in overdose (coma, convulsions, cardiac arrhythmias). Instead, SSRIs have become first-line agents for depression.

(4) **L**. Selegiline is a monoamine oxidase B inhibitor involved in the breakdown of dopamine. It is particularly useful when used in combination with levodopa therapy.

(5) **B**. The drug commonly added is either carbidopa or benserazide. These prevent peripheral conversion of levodopa to dopamine through inhibition of DOPA decarboxylase. This both reduces peripheral side-effects and increases cerebral availability of the drug.

Answer 20: MCQ

See *Medical Sciences at a Glance* (Defence against pathology).

(c) The toll-like receptors (TLRs) are a superfamily of receptors that are a core component of the innate immune response. They are predominantly found on resident macrophages and dendritic cells and react to a large variety of antigens that are harmful through humans. Activation of a TLR directly results in activation of dendritic cells and macrophages (c) which then indirectly stimulate a local immune response by secreting cytokines (d,e). By initiating macrophage activation, they initiate the first steps that eventually lead to antigen presentation but are not directly involved in antigen presentation or activation of T cells (a,b).

Answer 21: EMQ

See *Medical Pharmacology at a Glance*, **7th edn** (**Drugs used in angina, Poisoning**).

(1) **G**. The nitrate is metabolised to nitric oxide (NO) that activates guanylyl cyclase to increase cGMP. This in turn activates protein kinase G to cause vascular smooth muscle relaxation.

(2) **L**. Tetrodotoxin is found in a number of organisms including the puffer fish. It is used as an experimental agent.

(3) **H**. Lead paints used to be common in the past when lead poisoning was a major issue. Children of families moving into old homes with existing lead paint are occasionally seen in hospital. This is because lead paint can taste sweet, making ingestion more likely, but painters have also been known to present with lead poisoning following surface preparations such as sanding of walls, giving the condition the nickname 'painter's colic'.

(4) **B**. Botulinum toxin is particularly lethal. It prevents the release of acetylcholine at the neuromuscular junction. It is the ingestion of the toxin that is dangerous, not the bacteria or spores, except in infants. Honey ingestion can cause infantile botulism.

(5) **D**. This activation pathway leads to an increase in activity of the cystic fibrosis transmembrane regulator (CFTR), which is a chloride channel. The increased secretion of chloride leads to increased sodium and water loss, thereby giving profuse diarrhoea.

Answer 22: MCQ

See *Medical Pharmacology at a Glance*, **7th edn** (**Antipsychotic drugs**).

(d) The two major agents that cause gynaecomastia on the list are typical antipsychotics, e.g. haloperidol and the H_2 receptor antagonist cimetidine. Haloperidol is an antidopaminergic drug and therefore removes the dopaminergic inhibition of pituitary prolactin release, resulting in galactorrhoea. Haloperidol in this patient is likely to be used for schizophrenia, whereas there is no indication for cimetidine.

Answer 23: EMQ

See *Medical Pharmacology at a Glance*, **7th edn** (**Antiarrhythmic drugs**).

(1) **F**. Amiodarone is a class III antiarrhythmic which inhibits K^+ channels and slows repolarisation. It has many side-effects – pulmonary fibrosis, hepatic dysfunction and thyroid disease are among the most important.

(2) **B**. This requires you to know the common antiarrhythmics in each class. Class Ia: procainamide; class Ib: lidocaine; class II: propranolol; class III: sotalol, amiodarone; class IV: verapamil; class V: adenosine.

(3) **H**. The clinical vignette describes a supraventricular tachycardia. Adenosine stimulates A_1 receptors and acetylcholine-sensitive K^+ channels. It hyperpolarises the atrioventricular node and thereby inhibits conduction to the ventricles. It is extremely short acting with a half-life of approximately 10 sec.

(4) **E**. Rate-slowing drugs in atrial fibrillation are calcium channel blockers (verapamil and diltiazem), β-adrenergic receptor

blockers and digoxin. β-blockers have the potential to worsen asthma. β-blockers should not worsen COPD and actually have been shown to have a mortality benefit.

(5) **C**. Thyroid hormone increases β-adrenergic receptor action and therefore β-blockers are most useful in this scenario.

Answer 24: MCQ

See *Medical Pharmacology at a Glance*, **7th edn** (**Drugs acting on the sympathetic system**).

(d) Selegiline is a monoamine oxidase B inhibitor. Cheese and red wine, which the person has likely been eating, contain high amounts of tyramine that is normally metabolised by monoamine oxidase inhibitors. Tyramine is an indirectly acting sympathomimetic. It has no sympathomimetic actions on its own but is taken up by the transport system into vesicles where it displaces noradrenaline and other neurotransmitters, first into the cytoplasm and then into the synapse. This can cause a malignant hypertension, as in this scenario.

Answer 25: SAQ

Drug monitoring requires a large service set-up and is very costly. As such, plasma concentration is only worthwhile when a given set of conditions is fulfilled. First, the effects need to be difficult to measure in clinical practice, such as with antiepileptic drugs or warfarin (1). The concentration in the blood needs to be critical for the drug's efficacy, as is illustrated by a target INR in which there is therapeutic benefit only for a narrow therapeutic range (2). There is patient variability and to achieve the same effect, different doses are needed in different patients (3). There also needs to be a clear target range that does not vary between patients (4). Finally, drug level monitoring needs to be accessible and quick enough to adjust dosing in time (5).

Answer 26: True/False

See *Medical Pharmacology at a Glance*, **7th edn** (**Drugs acting on the sympathetic system**).

(a) **True**. Noradrenaline will act on α_1-adrenergic receptors which are G-protein-coupled receptors ($G_{\alpha q}$), activating phospholipase C to break down PIP_2 to DAG and IP_3. IP_3 acts on IP_3 receptors, which are Ca^{2+} channels on the sarcoplasmic reticulum, resulting in calcium release.

(b) **False**. α_2-Adrenergic receptors act presynaptically to inhibit noradrenaline release, i.e. they provide negative feedback.

(c) **False**. Propranolol is a non-selective β-blocker. Although β_2-adrenergic receptors can be found on vascular smooth muscle, they act to cause vasodilation. Propranolol has very minimal effect on peripheral vascular resistance.

(d) **True**. A decrease in diameter of blood vessels, primarily arterioles, increases total peripheral resistance and therefore increases blood pressure. Remember mean arterial pressure (MAP) is equal to cardiac output (CO) × total peripheral resistance (TPR): MAP = CO × TPR.

(e) **True**. Vasopressin (also called antidiuretic hormone) is indeed another vasoconstrictor agent used as a vasopressor.

Answer 27: SAQ

See *Medical Pharmacology at a Glance*, **7th edn**.
Ciprofloxacin is a cytochrome P450 system inhibitor and therefore reduces the metabolism of warfarin. INR is likely to go up.

Amiodarone decreases the clearance of digoxin and therefore increases the risk of toxicity. In addition, both drugs slow conduction through the AV node and together increase the risk of atrioventricular block.

Verapamil (Ca^{2+} channel blocker) and propranolol (β-blocker) are both negative inotropic and negative chronotropic drugs. Both reduce conduction through the AV node and therefore are contraindicated together due to risk of AV block, bradycardia and cardiac failure.

Isoniazid inhibits the cytochrome P450 system and therefore would increase the serum concentration of phenytoin. For example, suddenly stopping may lead to convulsions due to reduced phenytoin levels.

No effect. Rifampicin induces the hepatic cytochrome P450 system and interacts with a wide range of other drugs.

Answer 28: MCQ

See *Medical Pharmacology at a Glance*, 7th edn (Drugs acting on the gastrointestinal tract I: peptic ulcer) or *Medical Sciences at a Glance* (Upper GI physiology).

(a) *Helicobacter pylori* is a gram-negative rod that colonises the majority of duodenal and gastric ulcers. However, most individuals colonised with the bacteria do not develop a peptic ulcer. Treatment normally involves two antibiotics and a proton pump inhibitor. Sometimes metronidazole is used instead of amoxicillin or other antibiotics if there is resistance. Bismuth may also be added as 'quadruple therapy' under certain protocols.

Answer 29: SAQ

See *Medical Pharmacology at a Glance*, 7th edn (Drugs used in heart failure) or *Medical Sciences at a Glance* (Cardiovascular pathophysiology).

Diuretics, e.g. loop diuretics or thiazides – diuresis leading to reduction of preload.

Angiotensin converting enzyme inhibitors – reduced perfusion of the kidneys leads to activation of the renin-angiotensin-aldosterone system, causing fluid retention.

β-Blockers: inhibit the increased sympathetic stimulation of the heart seen in cardiac failure.

Aldosterone antagonists.

Digoxin: positive inotropic agent by inhibition of the Na$^+$/K$^+$ ATPase.

Answer 30: MCQ

See *Medical Pharmacology at a Glance*, 7th edn (Immunosuppressants and antirheumatoid drugs).

(a) Mycophenolate mofetil inhibits B and T cell proliferation by inhibition of inosine monophosphate dehydrogenase. This is the only way for B and T cells to synthesise purines, whereas other cells have an alternative pathway.

8 Pharmacology exam 2

Questions

Question 1: SAQ (5 points)
Pharmaceutical companies are continuously trying to develop new drugs to target diseases of the body. Name three different potential types of targets in humans and give an example drug class.

Question 2: MCQ
Antibiotic susceptibility testing is carried out on a urine sample. There is a clear area surrounding the disc labelled T (trimethoprim) but not around the disc labelled A (amoxicillin). What is the likely mechanism of resistance to the antibiotic?
(a) Methylation of 23S rRNA
(b) β-lactamase cleavage of β-lactam rings
(c) Phosphorylation of antibiotic
(d) DNA gyrase mutation
(e) Reduced uptake

Question 3: EMQ

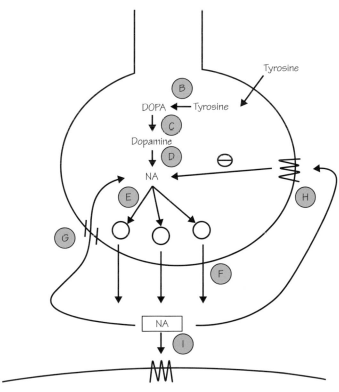

Figure 8.1 Noradrenergic nerve terminal.

For each of the scenarios below, choose the most appropriate answer from the figure above.
(1) A 26-year-old pregnant woman is diagnosed with pregnancy-induced hypertension. She is started on methyldopa. What is its main target in the figure above?

(2) A 19-year-old man presents to the emergency department with agitation and chest pain following the ingestion of cocaine. What part of the adrenergic transmission is affected by cocaine?
(3) A 45-year-old man who was diagnosed with a phaeo-chromocytoma presents with headache, tachycardia and hypertension. He is started on phenoxybenzamine. What is the site of action?
(4) A 44-year-old woman is started on amitriptyline for depression. What is its most important mechanism of action on adrenergic transmission in the context of its antidepressant action?
(5) A 76-year-old woman with confusion and a blood pressure of 240/140 is treated with IV guanethidine, a drug licensed for this purpose. What is its site of action?

Question 4: MCQ
A medical student is working in a lab on a drug named MJ867, which is an inverse agonist of the GABA$_A$ receptor. Which of the curves shown in Figure 8.2 represents the likely effect of the drug on the receptor action?

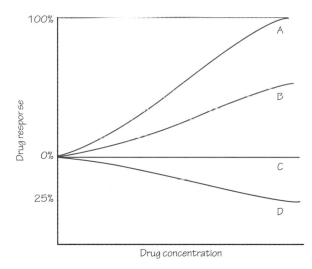

Figure 8.2 Graph showing different options of drug receptor action.

(a) A
(b) B
(c) C
(d) D
(e) None of the above

Question 5: EMQ
A Glomerulus
B Proximal convoluted tubule (PCT)
C Descending loop of Henle
D PCT and descending loop of Henle
E Thick ascending loop of Henle

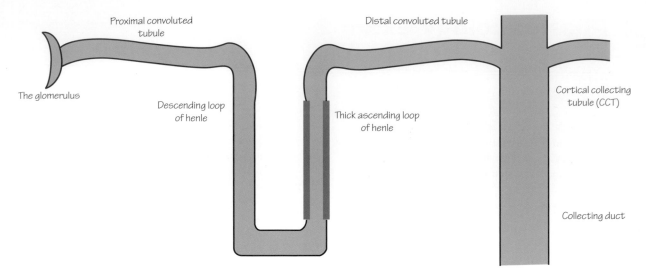

Figure 8.3 Kidney nephron.

F Distal convoluted tubule (DCT)
G Cortical collecting tubule (CCT)
H CCT and collecting duct

For each of the scenarios below, choose the most appropriate answer from the list above.
(1) A 34 year old admitted after a road traffic accident is found to have raised intracranial pressure and is treated immediately with an intravenous infusion of a diuretic. What is the primary site of action of this agent?
(2) In preparation to start climbing Everest, a medical student starts taking a carbonic anhydrase inhibitor. Where does this agent act?
(3) A 72-year-old man is admitted in decompensated heart failure after forgetting to take his diuretics for 3 weeks. The admitting physician decides to give a bolus injection of a diuretic. What is the site of action of the first-line diuretic used in acute heart failure?
(4) Hypokalaemia is a side-effect associated with the use of loop diuretics. Potassium-sparing diuretics may be used to reduce the complications. Where do they act?
(5) The first-line antihypertensive diuretic agent in all national and international guidelines acts at the … ?

Question 6: MCQ

A researcher has developed a new medication X acting on β-adrenergic receptors and compares it to already available compounds.

Which *one* of the following statements can be supported by the evidence from the graph in Figure 8.4?
(a) The new drug is an antagonist with a high affinity for the receptor.
(b) The new drug has greater potency than compound B.
(c) C is a competitive antagonist with regard to the new drug.
(d) The new drug exerts its effect through allostery.
(e) The new drug has lower affinity for the receptor than drug A.

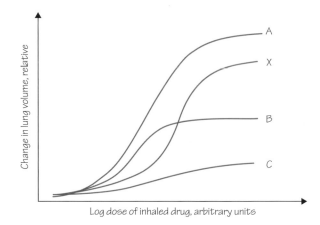

Figure 8.4 Graph of drug dosage against relative change in lung volume.

Question 7: MCQ

A patient on intensive care who has endocarditis receives vancomycin and flucloxacillin for 5 weeks. Which *one* of the following statements about vancomycin is true?
(a) Vancomycin inhibits the recycling of bactorenol phosphate to start a new round of peptidoglycan synthesis.
(b) Vancomycin cannot be given orally because it is a peptide that is broken down by the digestive system.
(c) Vancomycin resistance is now commonplace in infections with *Staphylococcus aureus*.
(d) Vancomycin resistance occurs predominantly due to the synthesis of bacterial peptidases that digest vancomycin.
(e) Vancomycin resistance poses an important problem in intensive care units.

Question 8: EMQ

A Atenelol
B Cholestyramine
C Clofibrate
D Ezetemibe
E Fish oil
F Nicotinic acid

G Orlistat

H Simvastatin

I Abstinence from alcohol

J Smoking cessation

For each of the scenarios below, choose the most appropriate answer from the list above.

(1) A 74-year-old man has marked hyperlipidaemia despite maximal dose statin therapy. His doctor considers adding a drug that inhibits lipid absorption by blocking a lipid transport protein. Which of the above fits this description?

(2) A smoker with a BMI of 37 who drinks 35 units of alcohol a week presents to his GP concerned about a family history of cardiovascular disease. Which one of the above interventions will have the largest impact on his cardiovascular risk?

(3) A 65-year-old man suffers a myocardial infarction. His LDL and total cholesterol are high. What secondary prevention should he be started on?

(4) A patient already takes a statin. Which other medication, when added, will markedly increase her risk of myositis?

(5) A 54-year-old obese man (BMI 40) has tried diet modification and regular exercise to lose weight without much success. His doctor describes a drug that would cause malabsorption and could help with weight loss. Choose the drug from the list above.

Question 9: SAQ (5 points)

Processes in the body that activate a signalling cascade also provide their off-switch. What are the cellular mechanisms by which sustained β-adrenoreceptor activation is controlled?

Question 10: MCQ

A patient with type II diabetes mellitus arrives at the clinic. His repeat blood pressure reading is again over 140/90. His GP considers an ACE inhibitor. Which one of the following statements is true about ACE inhibitors in this context?

(a) Renin concentration will decrease after administration of an ACE inhibitor.

(b) Bilateral renal artery stenosis is a contraindication to ACE inhibitors because they constrict the afferent arteriole.

(c) ACE inhibitors may cause a cough due to inhibition of bradykinin breakdown.

(d) ACE inhibitors may worsen the patient's glycaemic control.

(e) ACE inhibitors result in a chronic decline in renal function.

Question 11: SAQ (3 points)

Fill in the blanks with the most appropriate answer (½ point for each).

Dyspepsia can be targeted through various mechanisms. Inhibition of the (a) _____ on the luminal surface of gastric parietal cells prevents gastric acid secretion. Alternative options include inhibition of histamine-induced acid secretion by acting at (b) _____ receptors. Magnesium hydroxide is an (c)_____ that acts to (d) _____. (e)_____, a bacteria, is commonly found in the general population but is known to be involved in significant percentage of peptic ulcers. Treatment is with a combination of (f) _____.

Question 12: MCQ

A 17 year old with recurrent tonic clonic seizures is started on phenytoin. Which one of the following statements about phenytoin is true?

(a) It is an antagonist at the $GABA_A$ receptor.

(b) It is a first-line drug in status epilepticus.

(c) It is a type II antiarrhythmic in the Vaughan Williams classification.

(d) The mechanism for phenytoin excretion is easily saturated, resulting in a higher risk of toxicity.

(e) When therapeutic, phenytoin metabolism is proportional to its plasma concentration.

Question 13: MCQ

A patient who has an estimated GFR of 60 mL/min is given a 300 mg dose of gentamicin. The initial serum peak level is 6 μg/mL. Gentamicin is known to behave like inulin with regard to its renal excretion and is excreted by the kidneys only. It is only minimally bound to plasma proteins. Given the above information, calculate the clearance of gentamicin:

(a) 50 mL/min

(b) 60 mL/min

(c) 120 mL/min

(d) 240 mL/min

(e) 1800 mL/min

Question 14: True/False

A woman with congestive cardiac failure is started on intravenous furosemide. Which of the following statements is true?

(a) Furosemide acts within seconds to minutes in this scenario.

(b) Furosemide acts on the Na^+/K^+ exchanger in the loop of Henle.

(c) Furosemide is a sulphonamide.

(d) The main side-effect of furosemide is headache.

(e) Furosemide has no proven mortality benefit in this scenario.

Question 15: True/False

A patient takes twice-daily propranolol. It is known that propranolol has a high C^{bound}:C^{free} ratio. Which of the following statements about its pharmacokinetic properties are true?

(a) The high C^{bound}:C^{free} ratio aids delivery of the drug to tissues.

(b) The rate of absorption of oral propranolol will influence the steady-state concentration.

(c) The availability of propranolol if given orally will influence the steady-state concentration.

(d) A loading dose needs to be between four- and fivefold higher than the maintainance dose.

(e) Cytochrome P450 system inhibitors such as cimetidine and sulphonamides can increase the metabolism of various hepatically metabolised drugs.

Question 16: MCQ

A 17 year old is admitted after an impulsive paracetamol overdose. Which one of the following statements are true regarding paracetamol overdose?

(a) Paracetamol has no action on COX 1 or COX 2.

(b) The antidote to paracetamol poisoning is the administration of an essential amino acid.

(c) A metabolic acidosis is the main concenrn during poisoning and patients may require dialysis.

(d) Effects of poisoning manifest themselves within 4 h.

(e) Paracetamol is a potent anti-inflammatory.

Question 17: SAQ (5 points)

Parkinson's disease is due to loss of the dopaminergic neurons in the nitrostriatal pathway leading to a resting tremor, bradykinesia and rigidity. Discuss five classes of drugs used to target parkinsonism.

Question 18: MCQ

A patient complains of postoperative nausea. The junior doctor considers the various options available. Which one of the following statements about antiemetics is true?

(a) Domperidone does not cross the blood–brain barrier.

(b) Ondansetron is an antagonist at a G-protein-coupled receptor.

(c) Ondansetron acts to prevent nausea in the gastrointestinal tract where 90% of serotonin in the body is produced.

(d) Some antipsychotic medications act on the vomiting centre.

(e) Pharmacological treatment of nausea is more successful than that of vomiting.

Question 19: EMQ

A Ciprofloxacin
B Amoxicillin
C Polymyxins
D Vancomycin
E Gentamicin
F Trimethoprim
G Sulfamethoxazole
H Erythromycin

For each question below, choose the most appropriate antibiotic from the list above.

(1) Antibiotic administered orally for *Clostridium difficile* treatment which acts by binding to D-Ala-D-Ala, preventing peptidoglycan cross-linkage.

(2) A 19 year old presents with a 2-week history of sore throat, lethargy and lymphadenopathy. He is started on an antibiotic that mimics D-Ala-D-Ala and binds to the enzyme necessary for peptidoglycan cross-linkage. He soon returns with a rash.

(3) Antibiotic which binds to 30S ribosome unit causing errors in protein synthesis. It has poor oral bioavailability and poor action against anaerobes.

(4) A 72 year old, who is on regular warfarin, is treated for her urinary tract infection with a DNA gyrase inhibitor. Three days later she returns with a very high prothrombin time/INR.

(5) Bacteriostatic antibiotic which acts through binding to the 50S ribosome subunit and inhibiting protein synthesis. Used in respiratory tract infections to provide better coverage for atypical pneumonia over penicillins.

Question 20: MCQ

An anaesthetic consultant asks his junior resident to manage an anesthetised patient as the surgery is completed. The junior resident administers neostigmine to reverse the patient's paralysis for surgery. However, after administration of the agent no muscle activity is noticed. Which muscle relaxant was used?

(a) Acetylcholinesterase inhibitor

(b) Atropine

(c) Suxamethonium

(d) Tubocurare

(e) Botulinum toxin

(f) Bungarotoxin

Question 21: True/False

(a) Atropine has widespread action including inhibition of neuromuscular transmission.

(b) Nicotine administration would be expected to have an effect on parasympathetic and sympathetic pathways.

(c) Excess physostigmine would be expected to produce symptoms consistent with excess parasympathetic nervous system activation.

(d) Pilocarpine should be administered immediately during an asthma exacerbation in addition to salbutamol.

(e) Acetylcholine stimulates vascular dilation through action on the endothelium.

Question 22: SAQ (5 points)

A 52 year old has had multiple myocardial infarctions leading to congestive heart failure due to a reduced left ventricular ejection fraction. Name five classes of drugs that would be used in chronic heart failure.

Question 23: True/False

Which of the following are true regarding pharmacodynamics?

(a) Phenytoin observes zero-order elimination.

(b) Volume of distribution $= \dfrac{\text{amount of drug}}{\text{plasma drug concentration}}$.

(c) If chloroquine is highly lipophilic it will have a low volume of distribution and poor absorption.

(d) To increase the urinary elimination of a weak acid, use bicarbonate.

(e) In first-order elimination, the rate of drug removal is directly related to the drug concentration.

Question 24: MCQ

A 34-year-old man presents with a tachycardia of 150 bpm that is diagnosed as atrial fibrillation. He is given flecainide to attempt cardioversion. What is the mechanism for this action?

(a) Increases action potential and refractory period duration by K^+-channel blockade.

(b) Reduction of calcium currents through β-adrenoreceptor antagonism.

(c) Increases K^+ outflux, thus causing hyperpolarisation.

(d) Inhibition of voltage-gated Na^+ channels.

(e) Direct blockade of voltage-gated Ca^{2+} current.

Question 25: MCQ

A 55-year-old man in a coronary care unit is started on an inotrope infusion for symptomatic bradycardia that has failed to respond to atropine. The monitors register the following parameters during the infusion (Figure 8.5).

Which drug was most probably administered in this setting?

(a) Adrenaline

(b) Noradrenaline

(c) Dobutamine

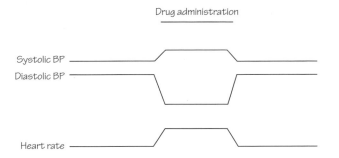

Drug administration
_____

Systolic BP _____
Diastolic BP _____

Heart rate _____

Figure 8.5 Systolic and diastolic blood pressure and heart rate before, during and after infusion of the inotrope.

(d) Isoprenaline
(e) Sotalol

Question 26: MCQ

A 22 year old is treated for acne vulgaris with oral tetracycline but without any improvement. Which *one* of the following can affect the action of tetracyclines?
(a) Concomitant use of calcium carbonate antacid.
(b) Phenytoin induces the cytochrome P450 system.
(c) Renal failure affects excretion.
(d) Congenital deficiency of activating enzyme.
(e) Treatment requires antivirals.

Question 27: EMQ

A Ranitidine
B Aluminium hydroxide
C Bismuth
D Omeprazole
E Lactulose
F Metoclopramide
G Infliximab
H Calcium carbonate
I Cyclizine
J Erythropoietin
K Misoprostol

For each of the descriptions below, choose the most appropriate answer from the list above.
(1) A proton pump inhibitor that may be used for the treatment of dyspepsia in a 32-year-old man.
(2) Used to treat a 43 year old with diabetic gastroparesis to improve motility. Contraindicated in mechanical gastrointestinal obstruction, and also used as an antiemetic.

(3) A 28-year-old woman in the first trimester who would like an abortion. Off-licence use includes cervical ripening and labor induction later in pregnancy.
(4) A 72-year-old woman who opens her bowels every 3–4 days uses an agent to increase the H_2O content of her stools to make them easier to pass.
(5) A 46 year old allergic to PPIs is prescribed a histamine receptor antagonist to reduce gastric acid production but subsequently suffers from vitamin B_{12} deficiency.

Question 28: MCQ

A medical student is studying the function of an enzyme. Which *one* of the following is correct?
(a) V_{max} is unrelated to the enzyme concentration.
(b) The lower the K_m, the higher the affinity.
(c) V_{max} is inversely related to the enzyme concentration.
(d) A competitive inhibitor decreases the K_m.
(e) A non-competitive inhibitor increases the K_m.

Question 29: MCQ

A patient is given a heart rate-slowing drug to treat a tachycardia. The patient has renal failure. Which of the following could accumulate in this patient and lead to dangerous AV nodal block?
(a) Digoxin
(b) Verapamil
(c) Captopril
(d) Spironolactone
(e) Heparin

Question 30: True/False

Which of the following is true regarding antiarrhythmic drugs that a physician has at her disposal?
(a) Vaughan Williams class IV drugs delay repolarisation by inhibition of K^+ channels.
(b) Digoxin treats atrial fibrillation by slowing atrioventricular conduction.
(c) Atropine is contraindicated in bradycardia and is potentially lethal.
(d) Daily adenosine is used for paroxysmal supraventricular tachycardia due to its effects on the AV node.
(e) Amiodarone, although a class III antiarrhythmic agent, has antiarrhythmic effects as a result of actions in addition to K^+ channel block.

Answers to Exam 2

Answer 1: SAQ

See *Medical Pharmacology at a Glance*, **7th edn (Introduction: principles of drug action)**.

Transporters: proton pump inhibitors inhibit the H^+/K^+ ATPase (reduces acid production in dyspepsia) – other examples include Na^+/K^+ ATPase inhibition, diuretics (Na^+/Cl^- co-transporter inhibition).

Ion channels: calcium channel antagonists used in hypertension, e.g. amlodipine.

Enzymes: angiotensin converting enzyme inhibitors, catechol-O-methyltransferase inhibitor, cyclo-oxygenase inhibition by non-steroidal anti-inflammatory drugs.

DNA synthesis: chemotherapy agents may not only affect enzymes involved in DNA synthesis but also damage DNA by mimicking purines/pyrimidines in DNA synthesis.

Microtubule action: microtubules are an essential part of the cytoskeleton. Examples include antigout medication.

Answer 2: MCQ

See *Medical Pharmacology at a Glance*, **7th edn (Antibacterial drugs that inhibit cell wall synthesis: penicillins, cephalosporins, and vancomycin)**.

(b) β-lactamase enzymes can cleave and inactivate β-lactam antibiotics, i.e. penicillins. To overcome this, β-lactamase inhibitors, e.g. clavulanic acid, may be administered with penicillins. Methylation of 23S rRNA (a) is typical of macrolide inhibition. Aminoglycosides may be inactivated by phosphorylation (c) or acetylation. Quinolones act through inhibition of DNA gyrase and mutations (d) can affect this action. Reduced uptake (e), e.g. through mutant porins, can affect several antibiotics, e.g. aminoglycosides, sulphonamides.

Answer 3: EMQ

See *Medical Pharmacology at a Glance*, **7th edn (Drugs acting on the sympathetic system)**.

(1) **H.** Methyldopa acts at the presynaptic terminals on α_2-adrenergic receptors, providing negative feedback for catecholamine release. Clonidine acts via the same mechanism.

(2) **G.** Cocaine inhibits the reuptake of norepinephrine by nerve terminals, in addition to its local anaesthetic effect through inhibition of sodium channels.

(3) **I.** Phenoxybenzamine is an irreversible α-adrenergic receptor inhibitor used to block the effect of high levels of circulating catecholamines.

(4) **G.** Amitriptyline, like other tricyclic antidepressants, acts on norepinephrine reuptake, thereby increasing norepinephrine transmission.

(5) **E.** Guanethidine previously was an important agent used in the treatment of hypertension. However, alternative agents are preferred these days. It is taken up into presynaptic vesicles, replacing norepinephrine and leading to a depletion of norepinephrine stores.

Answer 4: MCQ

See *Medical Pharmacology at a Glance*, **7th edn (Drug–receptor interactions)**.

(d) Inverse agonism refers to a drug that binds to a receptor and reduces its basal level of activity at resting state. That is, when the drug binds, it effectively causes an opposite response to the full (a) or partial (b) agonist. Although inverse agonists decrease basal activity, they are still *agonists,* i.e. they *activate* their receptor.

Answer 5: EMQ

See *Medical Pharmacology at a Glance*, **7th edn (Drugs acting on the kidney: diuretics)**.

(1) **D.** Mannitol is a polysaccharide that is freely filtered at the glomerulus but cannot be reabsorbed. This creates an osmotic effect, reducing H_2O reabsorption with effects throughout the nephron but primarily at the PCT and the descending loop of Henle.

(2) **B.** Carbonic anhydrase inhibitors, e.g. acetazolamide, act at the PCT to reduce bicarbonate reabsorption.

(3) **E.** Loop diuretics, e.g. furosemide, are powerful agents that act on $Na^+/K^+/2Cl^-$ co-transporters in the thick ascending loop of Henle to increase diuresis. If a loop diuretic is not sufficient, a thiazide diuretic may be used to supplement the diuretic effect.

(4) **H.** The primary site of action of potassium-sparing diuretics, including aldosterone antagonists and epithelial sodium channel inhibitors, is the CCT and collecting duct. They also have smaller effects on the distal convoluted tubule.

(5) **F.** The first-line agents are thiazide diuretics such as chlorthalidone. They have the strongest and most extensive evidence for long-term benefit and act through Na^+/Cl^- co-transporters in the DCT.

Answer 6: MCQ

See *Medical Pharmacology at a Glance*, **7th edn (Drug–receptor interactions)**.

(c) The most important step to realise is that the above graph is a dose–response curve so no inferences can be made about affinity (a,e) or receptor interactions (d). Although it is possible to make a statement about potency from this graph, the relative potency of the two compounds varies with concentration in this example (b). Answer (c) is indeed correct as although both C and X are likely partial agonists at the receptor, C would act like a competitive antagonist with respect to X if both were present, as C barely has a response.

Answer 7: MCQ

See *Medical Pharmacology at a Glance*, **7th edn (Antibacterial drugs that inhibit cell wall synthesis: penicillins, cephalosporins, and vancomycin)**.

(e) Vancomycin is a glycopeptide antibiotic that adheres to the D-alanyl-D-alanine moiety of bacterial peptidoglycan and prevents cross-linking of the pentapeptides. This significantly impairs the stability of the bacterial wall and renders the bacteria susceptible to death via osmotic lysis. Vancomycin is not involved in the recycling of bactorenol phosphate (a). Vancomycin can be administered orally *as well as* intravenously. When given orally, it can only be used to treat enteral infections because it is not absorbed from the gut, not because it is digested (b). Vancomycin resistance occurs predominantly via plasmids that result in synthesis of D-alanyl-D-lactate or D-alanyl-D-serine in place of the original peptide, thus decreasing the affinity for vancomycin (d). Vancomycin-resistant *Staphylococcus aureus* thankfully remains a rare occurrence (c). However, vancomycin-resistant enterococci (VRE) are now commonplace (up to 50% of isolates) in intensive care settings and in the community. Because patients on intensive care are susceptible to enterococcal infections, vancomycin resistance has become an important problem in this setting (e).

Answer 8: EMQ

See *Medical Pharmacology at a Glance*, 7th edn (Lipid-lowering drugs).
(1) **D**.
(2) **J**. Smoking cessation is the most important modifiable risk factor for cardiovascular disease. Alcohol in moderation increases HDL cholesterol and therefore reduces risk of cardiovascular disease but in excess (as in this case) causes adverse effects, increasing LDL cholesterol and reducing HDL.
(3) **II**. Statins have repeatedly demonstrated reduction in cardiovascular mortality and cardiovascular events by reduction of LDL cholesterol. Statins are HMG CoA reductase inhibitors. HMG CoA reductase is the rate-limiting step in hepatic cholesterol synthesis. The liver increases expression of LDL receptors, thus reducing circulating cholesterol.
(4) **C**. Fibrates and statins both pose a risk of myositis and rhabdomyolysis, and together increase the risk to 1–5%. They can also cause derangement of liver function.
(5) **G**. Orlistat inhibits lipase activity in the intestine, thereby preventing digestion of triglycerides to free fatty acids for absorption. Due to this mechanism, it also affects absorption of fat-soluble vitamins (i.e. A, D, E, K).

Answer 9: SAQ

See *Medical Pharmacology at a Glance*, 7th edn (Introduction: principles of drug action).
The β-adrenoreceptor is a G-protein-coupled receptor and its activation results in a signalling cascade, leading to the activation of adenylate cyclase, production of cAMP and activation of PKA and its effector functions (1). The process is deactivated at multiple points. The α subunit of G_s has an intrinisic GTPase activity, resulting in its self-inactivation (2). PKA phosphorylates and activates phosphodiesterase and results in a decrease in cAMP concentration (3). PKA also activates β-adrenergic receptor kinase (βARK), which results in phosphorylation of the β-adrenoreceptor (4). β-Arrestin binds to the site of phosphorylation and causes homologous desensitisation (5) and targets the receptor for internalisation (6).

Answer 10: MCQ

See *Medical Pharmacology at a Glance*, 7th edn (Drugs used in hypertension).
(c) Angiotensin converting enzyme inhibitors are used to control hypertension in diabetic patients for a number of reasons. They have an effect on blood pressure by inhibiting the renin-angiotensin system. They act downstream of renin and thus there is a rise in renin concentrations due to reduced negative feedback (a). However, in addition to inhibiting ACE, they also inhibit breakdown of bradykinin which can lead to cough and sometimes angio-oedema. Both are indications for switching to an angiotensin receptor blocker. In bilateral renal artery stenosis, there is an appropriate rise in renin and aldosterone levels that causes hypertension which is necessary to perfuse the kidneys. Angiotensin inhibits this appropriate response of the axis (b). ACE inhibitors may actually improve glycaemic control or are at least neutral in that regard, and are thus preferable to β-blockers or thiazide diuretics in the diabetic patient (d). ACE inhibitors can cause an *acute* fall in renal function, but slow chronic renal decline in diabetic illness (e). Much of the benefit on kidney function probably arises from better blood pressure control, but other mechanisms have been postulated.

Answer 11: SAQ

See *Medical Pharmacology at a Glance*, 7th edn (Drugs acting on the gastrointestinal tract I: peptic ulcer).
(a) H^+/K^+ ATPase
(b) H_2-histamine
(c) Antacid
(d) Neutralise acid
(e) *Helicobacter pylori*
(f) Triple therapy (two antibiotics and a PPI)

Answer 12: MCQ

See *Medical Pharmacology at a Glance*, 7th edn (Antiepileptic drugs).
(d) Phenytoin binds to and stabilises the inactive state of the sodium channel (a). Even in the therapeutic range, phenytoin follows zero-order kinetics, resulting in a constant plasma metabolism (e) that does not correlate with the plasma concentration unlike most other drugs. It is because of this that small changes in dosing may result in amounts of phenytoin that cannot be excreted and build up with time, causing toxicity (d). It is used in status epilepticus if benzodiazepines have failed (b). It also has other applications and is rarely used as an antiarrhythmic. It is classified as a type I antiarrhythmic in the Vaughan Williams classification (c). Type II antiarrhythmics are β-blockers.

Answer 13: MCQ

See *Medical Pharmacology at a Glance*, 7th edn (Drug absorption, distribution and excretion).
(b) The question contains a mix of relevant and irrelevant information that has been intentionally included to confuse the examinee. We know that inulin is a small molecule that is freely filtered by the kidneys and neither reabsorbed nor secreted. Assuming the above for gentamicin, we know that the rate of excretion for gentamicin is equal to the eGFR multiplied by the concentration of free gentamicin. Clearance is the rate of excretion divided by the total concentration and thus clearance can be expressed as $CL = GFR \times \frac{C^{free}}{C^{total}}$. Because $C^{free} = C^{total}$ in this example, the clearance is equal to the GFR.

Answer 14: True/False

See *Medical Pharmacology at a Glance*, 7th edn (Drugs acting on the kidney: diuretics, Drugs used in heart failure).
(a) **True**. Furosemide, apart from its diuretic action, has another major mode of action. It acts as a vasodilator particularly to decrease preload. This action serves to improve pulmonary oedema and starts within minutes of intravenous administration.

(b) **False**. Furosemide acts on the $Na^+/K^+/2Cl^-$ channel in the thick ascending limb of the loop of Henle.

(c) **True**. Furosemide is an altered sulfa drug that was created when the diuretic properties of sulphonamides were accidentally discovered.

(d) **False**. The main side-effects of furosemide are hyponatraemia, acute kidney injury and orthostatic hypotension.

(e) **True**. This is contested, but as yet there is no proven mortality benefit of furosemide therapy in both chronic and decompensated cardiac failure (Evidence grade C). There are, however, ethical issues precluding randomised controlled trials as loop diuretics are often deemed necessary in the treatment of patients hospitalised with congestive cardiac failure and there is a definite symptomatic benefit.

Answer 15: True/False

See *Medical Pharmacology at a Glance*, 7th edn (**Drug metabolism, Drug absorption, distribution and excretion**).

(a) **True**. A high $C^{bound}:C^{free}$ ratio, i.e. a large proportion of medication bound to plasma and extracellular tissues, does aid delivery of a medication. This is particularly important for propranolol which binds very strongly.

(b) **False**. The rate of absorption does not affect the steady-state concentration if the bioavailability remains unchanged. To achieve steady-state concentration, it does thus not matter if a medication is given IV or orally, as long as the availability does not change. This certainly holds true for propranolol which is essentially fully absorbed via the oral route.

(c) **True**. The availability of propranolol does influence the steady-state concentration, as it is the fraction of the drug that reaches the circulation. The rest is lost in the gastrointestinal tract.

(d) **False**. For any drug with any dosing interval, it will take 4–5 half-lives to reach steady state by clinical convention (97% of steady-state level, in fact). However, this does not mean that a loading dose will equal four doses, as the loading dose depends on the volume of distribution.

(e) **False**. Inhibitors of the cytochrome P450 system increase the activity of various drugs, e.g. theophylline, warfarin, carbamazepine, but inhibit their metabolism. Thus caution must be used when combining such agents.

Answer 16: MCQ

See *Medical Pharmacology at a Glance*, 7th edn (**Poisoning**).
(b) Paracetamol (called acetaminophen in the USA) is an atypical NSAID that does have some selective action on COX 2 receptors, although its main mode of action and selectivity for the central nervous system are not fully understood and may involve COX 3 inhibition (a). It is a potent antipyretic, but has no inflammatory action (e). Paracetamol poisoning is a common and important clinical problem. The main concern is the delayed hepatotoxicity, which often manifests 12 h after the ingestion of the dose and may result in fulminant hepatic failure requiring transplantation (c, d). Treatment is by replenishing glutathione stores, which acts as a scavenger in these situations, and this can be done via methionine orally or N-acetylcysteine intravenously (b).

Answer 17: SAQ

See *Medical Pharmacology at a Glance*, 7th edn (**Drugs used in Parkinson's disease**).
Levodopa/carbidopa: levodopa is the precursor for dopamine synthesis. Dopamine does not penetrate the blood–brain barrier and cannot be directly administered. Carbidopa is a dopa decarboxylase inhibitor which prevents peripheral conversion of levodopa to dopamine.

Dopamine agonist. Like levodopa they act at the dopamine receptor, but their effects are less spectacular in return for less motor side effects.

Monoamine oxidase B inhibitor: inhibition of dopamine breakdown.

Catechol-O-methyltransferase inhibitor: inhibits dopamine breakdown.

Anticholinergics, e.g. benztropine – mainly effective in treating the tremor.

Amantadine: formerly used in influenza treatment, it has mild antiparkinsonian effects.

Answer 18: MCQ

See *Medical Pharmacology at a Glance*, 7th edn (**Drugs used in nausea and vertigo (antiemetics)**).
(a) Pharmacological treatment of nausea is more challenging than that of vomiting which is much easier to control using medication (e). Most antiemetics, including phenothiazine antipsychotics and ondansetron, have their predominant effect on the chemoreceptor trigger zone in the CNS, from which impulses are passed on to the vomiting centre (c,d). Although most serotonin receptors are 7-transmembrane receptors that are coupled to G-proteins, HT_3-receptors that are antagonised by ondansetron are ligand-gated ion channels, which are permeable to sodium, potassium and calcium ions (b). Domperidone is a D_2 antagonist that, unlike metoclopramide, does not cross the blood–brain barrier, resulting in fewer extrapyramidal side-effects.

Answer 19: EMQ

See *Medical Pharmacology at a Glance*, 7th edn (**Antibacterial drugs that inhibit cell wall synthesis: penicillins, cephalosporins and vancomycin, Antibacterial drugs that inhibit nucleic acid synthesis: sulphonamides, trimethoprim, quinolones and nitroimidazoles**).

(1) **D**. The two first-line drug treatments are metronidazole and vancomycin. Metronidazole is a drug precursor that is metabolised into cytotoxic compounds, causing DNA damage. It can be administered intravenously or orally in *C. difficile* treatment. Vancomycin is only administered orally for *C. difficile* treatment as it is not absorbed into the blood and remains within the GI tract.

(2) **B**. Infectious mononucleosis is caused by the Epstein–Barr virus and often is called kissing disease due to transmission via saliva between young adults experiencing a new relationship. Amoxicillin and ampicillin are contraindicated as they cause a rash in up to 90% of patients. The mechanism remains poorly defined.

(3) **E**. Gentamicin is an aminoglycoside and like all aminoglycosides has poor bioavailability. Its uptake is an oxygen-dependent active process.

(4) **A**. Ciprofloxacin is a quinolone which acts by inhibiting DNA gyrase, an enzyme responsible for negative supercoiling. It is a cytochrome p450 system inhibitor. Erythromycin,

sulphonamides and isoniazid are other antibiotics that act as inhibitors.

(5) **H**. Atypical pneumonias can be caused by mycoplasma, legionella and chlamydia. These are better treated with macrolides.

Answer 20: MCQ

See *Medical Pharmacology at a Glance*, 7th edn (**Drugs acting at the neuromuscular junction**).

(c) Acetylcholine is the neurotransmitter released at the neuromuscular junction and broken down by acetylcholinesterase. Neostigmine inhibits this enzyme (a) and is used to increase the acetylcholine concentration at the neuromuscular junction to reverse the actions of a competitive neuromuscular junction blocker such as tubocurare (d). Botulinum toxin (e) blocks SNARE proteins at the prejunctional terminal, preventing exocytosis of the neurotransmitter, ACh. It is used clinically in local areas such as for cosmetic purposes and achalasia. Suxamethonium (c) is a depolarising non-competitive blocker used as a muscle relaxant in anaesthetics and therefore is not affected by an agent that increases acetylcholine concentration.

Answer 21: True/False

See *Medical Pharmacology at a Glance*, 7th edn (**Autonomic drugs acting at cholinergic synapses**).

(a) **False**. There are two major groups of acetylcholine receptors peripherally: nicotinic and muscarinic receptors. Atropine acts on muscarinic receptors and therefore does not have an effect at the neuromuscular junction where nicotinic acetylcholine receptors are found.

(b) **True**. This requires you to remember that nicotinic acetylcholine receptors are found at the autonomic nervous system postganglionic neurons.

(c) **True**. Physostigmine is an acetylcholinesterase inhibitor which increases acetylcholine levels at the synapses and effects would include bradycardia, sweating, lacrimation and pupillary constriction.

(d) **False**. Pilocarpine is a muscarinic agonist and is clinically found only as eye drops for glaucoma. A muscarinic agonist would cause further bronchoconstriction. Instead, a muscarinic antagonist, e.g. ipratropium, would be useful in this situation in addition to a β-adrenergic agonist such as salbutamol.

(e) **True**. Acetylcholine acts on vascular endothelial cells to stimulate nitric oxide release that act on neighbouring smooth muscle cells through the cGMP pathway.

Answer 22: SAQ

Angiotensin converting enzyme inhibitors, e.g. captopril (suffix–pril): long-term effect due to reduced ventricular remodelling.

β-adrenergic receptor blockers, e.g. metoprolol, carvedilol: negative chronotropic and inotropic agent and therefore cardiac workload and action of an overactive sympathetic nervous system.

Loop diuretics, e.g. furosemide: by causing diuresis, prevent volume overload which would place the patient at a non-optimum position on the curve described by the Frank–Starling law of the heart.

Aldosterone antagonist/potassium-sparing diuretic, e.g. spironolactone.

Digoxin: positive inotropic agent that inhibits sarolemmal Na^+/ K^+ ATPase. This increases intracellular Na^+ which reduces the removal of cytoplasmic Ca^{2+} by the Na^+/Ca^{2+} exchanger. Digoxin does not have a mortality benefit but has been demonstrated to reduce hospitalisation.

Thiazide diuretic, e.g. metolazone: thiazide diuretics are not commonly used for congestive heart failure except in patients where loop diuretics are not sufficient to prevent volume overload.

Answer 23: True/False

See *Medical Pharmacology at a Glance*, 7th edn (**Drug absorption, distribution and excretion**).

(a) **True**. In zero-order elimination, the rate of elimination does not vary with concentration, i.e. the amount of drug eliminated is constant. Ethanol also demonstrates zero-order elimination.

(b) **True**. A low volume of distribution indicates that the drug distributes mainly in blood. Drugs that distribute in extracellular space and tissues have high volumes.

(c) **False**. Chloroquine is highly lipophilic and as a result is sequestered in adipose tissue in the body. This gives it a volume of distribution >10,000 L.

(d) **True**. One example is salicylate. Polar (ionised) species become trapped. A weak acid will be trapped if the pH is alkaline. Conversely, weak bases should be treated with ammonium chloride to make the environment acidic.

(e) **True**. This means that a constant fraction (as compared to constant amount in zero-order elimination) of drug is eliminated for a given amount of time. Therefore, in first-order elimination the amount of drug eliminated will progressively decrease with time.

Answer 24: MCQ

See *Medical Pharmacology at a Glance*, 7th edn (**Antiarrhythmic drugs**).

(d) Flecainide is a class Ic drug in the Singh Vaughan Williams classification. Like all class I drugs, it is a Na^+-channel antagonist affecting the rapid upstroke of the cardiomyocyte action potential. It demonstrates use dependency, i.e. the effect on the channels is higher at higher heart rates. Class II drugs are β-adrenoceptor blockers useful as a negative chronotropic agent in tachycardias, including fast atrial fibrillation (b). K^+-channel antagonists, e.g. amiodarone (a), are class III agents that are also used for cardioversion and often used if other agents fail. Class IV agents are calcium channel inhibitors that reduce conduction velocity and prolong the refractory period and PR interval (e). Adenosine acts via its own receptors leading to an increase in K^+ outflux (c).

Answer 25: MCQ

See *Medical Pharmacology at a Glance*, 7th edn (**Autonomic nervous system**).

(d) Isoprenaline, now only rarely used in clinical practice for resistant bradycardia where pacing is not available, best fits the graph above as it causes a fall in mean arterial pressure and tachycardia (d). It is a non-selective β-adrenergic agonist with hardly any action on α-receptors. Noradrenaline would raise systolic and diastolic blood pressure and cause a reflex bradycardia (b), whereas adrenaline would cause a similar picture as above but with a rise in mean arterial pressure (c). Dobutamine is a selective $β_1$-agonist, which would cause predominantly a tachycardia with little effect on blood pressure. Sotalol is a β-blocker with type III antiarrhythmic properties and would cause a fall in heart rate.

Answer 26: MCQ

See *Medical Pharmacology at a Glance*, **7th edn (Antibacterial drugs that inhibit protein synthesis: aminoglycosides, tetracyclines, macrolides and chloramphenicol).**

(a) *Propionibacterium acnes* is involved in the pathology of acne vulgaris. Tetracycline absorption is affected by antacids, especially Ca^{2+} containing but also aluminium and magnesium. Dairy products may also affect bioavailability of tetracycline, and tetracycline administration should be at least 1 h from meals.

Answer 27: EMQ

See *Medical Pharmacology at a Glance*, **7th edn (Drugs acting on the gastrointestinal tract I: peptic ulcer).**

(1) **D**. PPIs inhibit the H^+-K^+ ATPase required for gastric acid production.

(2) **F**. Metoclopramide is a D_2 dopaminergic receptor antagonist with secondary effects on serotonergic and muscarinic receptors mediating its antiemetic and prokinetic effects.

(3) **K**. Misoprostol as prostaglandin E1 is also used to prevent NSAID-induced gastric ulcers. In its role as an abortifacient, it is used in combination with other agents to expel the conceptus. It may be also used for cervical dilation before surgical removal.

(4) **E**. Lactulose is a non-digestible disaccharide, drawing water into the bowel due to its osmotic effect.

(5) **A**. With the advent of PPIs, H_2-receptor antagonists have become second-line agents used for peptic ulcer disease. It also affects gastric intrinsic factor release which is essential for the absorption of vitamin B_{12} by the terminal ileum.

Answer 28: MCQ

See *Medical Pharmacology at a Glance*, **7th edn (Drug–receptor interactions).**

(b) The Michaelis constant (K_m) is the substrate concentration where the reaction rate is half-maximum. Therefore, the lower the K_m, the higher the affinity. The presence of a competitive inhibitor increases the K_m without changing the V_{max} whereas a non-competitive inhibitor decreases the V_{max} and leaves the K_m unchanged.

Answer 29: MCQ

See *Medical Pharmacology at a Glance*, **7th edn (Antiarrhythmic drugs).**

(a) Digoxin prolongs the refractory period of the atrioventricular node through activation of the vagal nerve. It is renally excreted and can accumulate in the patient described. Of the other drugs listed, only verapamil, a calcium channel blocker, is a heart rate-slowing drug.

Answer 30: True/False

See *Medical Pharmacology at a Glance*, **7th edn (Antiarrhythmic drugs).**

(a) **False**. This requires knowledge of the Vaughan Williams classification: I Na^+ channel block (divided further into Ia, Ib, Ic); II β-adrenoceptor blockers, III K^+ channel blockers and IV Ca^{2+} channel blockers.

(b) **True**. Digoxin, a cardiac glycoside, increases vagal activity. Therefore, in AF digoxin does not affect the atrial dysrhythmia but by prolonging the atrioventricular conduction, it reduces the ventricular contraction rate. This improves ventricular filling and thus stroke volume. It is a second-line agent for AF.

(c) **False**. Atropine, an antimuscarinic agent, is the first-line treatment in unstable bradycardia.

(d) **False**. Adenosine acts on A_1-receptors to block conduction through the AV node. It is administered intravenously and has a duration of action of less than 30 sec due to rapid metabolisation. Thus it is used in an emergency to terminate supraventricular tachycardia but serves no purpose in long-term treatment.

(e) **True**. Amiodarone acts on K^+, Na^+ and Ca^{2+} channels. It inhibits cardiac repolarisation via K^+ channel inhibition and prolongs the action potential. This also prolongs the QT interval.

9 Pathology exam 1

Questions

Question 1: MCQ

A 50-year-old obese man presents with a long history of lower chest discomfort. The results from a lower oesophageal biopsy read: 'Columnar epithelium containing goblet cells. No evidence of abnormal anisocytosis, poikilocytosis, hyperchromatic nuclei or mitotic figures'. What process has his oesophageal mucosa undergone?
(a) Hyperplasia
(b) Dysplasia
(c) Metaplasia
(d) Hypertrophy
(e) Phagocytosis

Question 2: MCQ

A 46-year-old heavy smoker and a long history of hypertension presents with crushing chest pain that is diagnosed as myocardial infarction. What is the most likely major pathological event that initiated the MI?
(a) Fibrous plaque expansion with accumulation of lipids and leucocytes leading to complete vascular obstruction
(b) Vasospasm near an atherosclerotic plaque
(c) Sudden plaque rupture with platelet aggregation and thrombus formation
(d) Cardiomyocyte coagulation necrosis with loss of cross-striations and nuclei fragmentation
(e) Neutrophil infiltration, hypercalcaemia and hypercontraction of myofibrils

Question 3: True/False

A 51 year old presents with severe abdominal pain and is found to have superior mesenteric artery occlusion on imaging. The patient undergoes surgery with resection of part of the small intestine. Determine whether the following are histological signs of irreversible cell injury that may be seen by the pathologist.
(a) Clumping of nuclear chromatin
(b) Cell membrane blebs
(c) Nuclear pyknosis
(d) Mitochondrial swelling
(e) Rupture of lysosomes

Question 4: SAQ (5 points)

A 12 year old receives a cut to his forearm while playing basketball. It initially builds and then immediately a clot forms. Describe the process of clot formation after activation of the extrinsic pathway.

Question 5: MCQ

A medical student returns from an elective in Uganda. She presents to her physician with cyclic fevers, dark urine, lethargy and jaundice. Which one of following is correct about malaria?
(a) *Plasmodium vivax* infection is the most severe.
(b) The transmission vector is the female tsetse fly.

(c) Malaria is caused by extracellular parasites targeting hepatocytes and erythrocytes.
(d) After infection of an erythrocyte, division occurs in the trophozoite stage.
(e) All of the above.

Question 6: EMQ

A HTLV-1
B Hepatitis B virus
C Hepatitis A virus
D Epstein–Barr virus
E Human papilloma virus
F Human herpes virus-8
G Human immunodeficiency virus
H Cytomegalovirus
I Merkel cell polyomavirus

Choose the most appropriate oncogenic virus for the scenarios below.
(1) A 24 year old with known acquired immunodeficiency syndrome presents with multiple purplish patches spread throughout the body.
(2) A 38-year-old woman is found to have cervical epithelial dysplasia on biopsy. She has been sexually active since the age of 21.
(3) A 12-year-old African boy presents with a B cell lymphoma found to have translocation 8;14.
(4) A 54 year old presents with a 7-month history of weight loss and anorexia. On examination, he is found to have a nodular liver and jaundice. The only other significant history is a blood transfusion 20 years ago.
(5) A 43-year-old man presenting with left-sided ear pain and cervical lymphadenopathy is diagnosed with nasopharyngeal carcinoma.

Question 7: MCQ

A 42 year old presents with a 3-week history of blood-stained sputum, night sweats and weight loss. A chest radiograph demonstrates lesions in the upper lung and hilar lymphadenopathy and the biopsy report reads: 'caseous granulomous necrosis seen'. Which of the following would be most helpful for the diagnosis?
(a) Antinuclear antibodies (ANA)
(b) Acid-fast stain
(c) Serum ACE
(d) CT chest
(e) Congo red stain

Question 8: SAQ (5 points)

Cell growth and differentiation play an important role in normal organ function and disregulation of this process can lead to pathology. For each of the following, provide a definition, indicate if the process is reversible or not and give an example of each: hyperplasia, dysplasia, anaplasia, neoplasia, hypertrophy.

Question 9: True/False

A 56 year old with HIV/AIDS presents to the emergency department feeling unwell. Which of the following is true regarding HIV/AIDS?

(a) HIV binds to CD4 and CXCR4 on T cells, and CD4 and CCR5 on macrophages.

(b) The virus contains single-stranded RNA that is used to synthesise double-stranded DNA to integrate into the host genome.

(c) HIV can only be transmitted to the child during delivery but not during pregnancy or breastfeeding.

(d) Acquired immunodeficiency syndrome describes the condition of a successful HIV infection.

(e) HAART refers to HIV/AIDS treatment consisting of at least two classes of antiretrovirals and at least three agents.

Question 10: MCQ

A 4-year-old girl receives a laceration to her foot while playing with friends. The area undergoes acute inflammation with rubor, dolor, calor and tumor. What mechanism is involved during this process?

(a) Neutrophil rolling mediated by selectins binding to sialyl Lewis^X.

(b) Formation of multinucleated giant cells due to macrophage activation.

(c) Decreased vascular permeability to reduce haemorrhage.

(d) Secretion of growth factors and fibrogenic cytokines for fibroblast stimulation.

(e) VEGF-mediated neutrophil tight binding on vascular endothelium.

Question 11: MCQ

A 53-year-old man presents with severe pain in the right knee which is warm, tender and painful on movement. The physician takes a joint fluid sample that shows neutrophils and polarised light microscopy demonstrates needle-shaped crystals that are negatively birefringent. What is the underlying condition?

(a) Gout
(b) Septic arthritis
(c) Pseudogout
(d) Rheumatoid arthritis
(e) Trauma

Question 12: SAQ (5 points)

The improvement of public health requires control of disease transmission. Name five different modes of viral transmission and provide an example of a virus.

Question 13: MCQ

A 56-year-old man who was diagnosed with multiple myeloma 8 months ago presents with shortness of breath secondary to diastolic heart failure and renal impairment. Renal biopsy demonstrates apple green birefringence on Congo red stain under polarised light. Which of the following is involved in the disease process?

(a) Anti-basement membrane antibodies

(b) IgG paraprotein
(c) AL amyloid
(d) Transthyretin
(e) α-Fetoprotein

Question 14: EMQ

A DiGeorge syndrome
B Bruton's agammaglobulinaemia
C Chediak–Higashi disease
D Chronic granulomatous disease
E Common variable immunodeficiency
F Splenectomy
G C9 complement deficiency
H IL-12 deficiency
I Job syndrome
J Wiskott–Aldrich syndrome

For each of the scenarios below, choose an answer from the list above.

(1) Recurrent viral and fungal infections due to T cell deficiency and associated with hypoparathyroidism and cardiac defects.

(2) Susceptibility to infections from encapsulated organisms, e.g. meningococcus, pneumococcus, *Haemophilus influenzae* type b.

(3) Defect in phagocyte respiratory burst due to impaired NADPH oxidase activity.

(4) Decreased mature B cell production and therefore decreased antibody production. X-linked recessive disorder associated with recurrent infections after 6 months.

(5) An impairment in phagocyte response due to a defect in microtubular polymerisation and impaired lysosomal emptying into phagosomes. Leads to recurrent pyogenic infections.

Question 15: MCQ

A 52-year-old woman who came off a flight 1 day ago presents with left calf swelling that is diagnosed as deep vein thrombosis. Which of the following falls within Virchow's triad?

(a) Prosthetic device that causes endothelial damage
(b) Nephrotic syndrome associated with hypercoagulability
(c) Venous stasis secondary to immobilisation
(d) Malignancy associated with hypercoagulability
(e) All of the above

Question 16: SAQ (5 points)

A 43-year-old man has a ST elevation myocardial infarction secondary to plaque rupture in the left circumflex artery. List five complications that may occur after a myocardial infarction and discuss the pathophysiology.

Question 17: MCQ

A 42-year-old woman presents with fatigue, dyspnoea (shortness of breath) and decreased urine output within the last 24 h. She has had diarrhoea over the past 5 days and abdominal cramps. Laboratory tests reveal decreased platelet counts and abnormal kidney function and her blood film shows features similar to those shown in Figure 9.1.

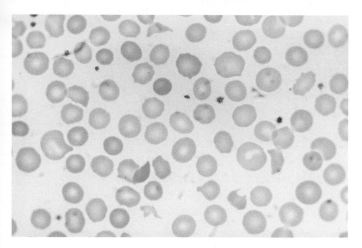

Figure 9.1 Results from peripheral blood smear. Image reproduced with permission from Bain BJ (2006) *Blood Cells: A Practical Guide*, 4th edn. Oxford: Wiley-Blackwell.

The most likely diagnosis is:
(a) iron deficiency
(b) renal failure
(c) glucose-6-phosphate dehydrogenase deficiency
(d) lead poisoning and sideroblastic anaemia
(e) haemolytic-uraemic syndrome,

Question 18: EMQ
A β-Thalassaemia
B Sickle cell anaemia
C Acute lymphoblastic leukaemia
D Acute myeloid leukaemia
E Chronic myelogenous leukaemia
F Chronic lymphocytic leukaemia
G Hodgkin lymphoma
H Burkitt lymphoma
I Follicular lymphoma

For each of the following scenarios, choose the most appropriate answer from the list above.
(1) A 50 year old presents with fatigue, malaise and weight loss over several months. Peripheral smear demonstrates neutrophilia, metamyelocytes, basophilia and eosinophilia. Genetic testing demonstrates t9:22, bcr-abl fusion.
(2) A 34-year-old woman presents with a 3-month history of enlarged, non-tender cervical lymph nodes. Biopsy demonstrates binucleated large cells that are CD[30+] positive consistent with Reed–Sternberg cells.
(3) On routine laboratory tests, a 72-year-old woman is found to have a white cell count of 34×10^9/L (normal range $4–11 \times 10^9$/L). On examination, she has hepatosplenomegaly, and peripheral blood smear demonstrates increased smudge cells.
(4) A 34-year-old man presents with shortness of breath, fatigue and fevers. Bone marrow biopsy demonstrates myeloblasts with Auer rods. Treatment is initiated with all-trans retinoic acid.
(5) A patient presents with B cell lymphoma demonstrating an indolent course and characterised by t14:18 translocation with bcl-2 activation.

Question 19: MCQ
A 3-year-old boy is brought into the emergency room with facial and tongue swelling, and stridor which started soon after pillow fighting with his older brother. He has had a long history of unexplained abdominal pain. What is the likely pathology?
(a) Adenine deaminase deficiency
(b) C1 esterase deficiency
(c) NADPH oxidase deficiency
(d) ADAMTS13 deficiency
(e) Glucose-6-phosphatase deficiency

Question 20: MCQ
A 34-year-old man is admitted with abdominal pain and is found to have abnormal liver function tests. The liver biopsy report reads: 'hepatocyte swelling and necrosis, Mallory bodies are seen within hepatocytes, and sinusoidal and perivenular fibrosis is seen'. What is the most likely cause?
(a) Chronic hepatitis C
(b) Acetaminophen/paracetamol overdose
(c) Alcoholic hepatitis
(d) Hereditary haemochromatosis
(e) Hepatic artery occlusion

Question 21: EMQ
A Osteoarthritis
B Rheumatoid arthritis
C Septic arthritis
D Pseudogout
E Gout
F Osteoporosis
G Paget's disease
H Metastatic cancer
I Primary hyperparathyroidism
J Osteomalacia
K Vitamin D intoxication

For each of the following scenarios, choose the most appropriate answer from the list above.
(1) A 52-year-old man with a history of hypertension presents to the emergency department with an inflamed tender right knee joint. Joint aspiration identifies needle shaped crystals that are negatively birefringent on polarised light microscopy.
(2) A 73 year old with a history of vertebral and right hip fractures is found to have decreased bone mineral density on DEXA scan.
(3) A 53-year-old ex-football player with a history of knee injuries in his 20s presents with a several-year history of progressively worsening right knee pain. Radiography of the joint demonstrates loss of joint space, subchondral cyst formation and osteophytes.
(4) A 34-year-old woman presents with a several-month history of bone pain and reports that she was recently treated for nephrolithiasis (kidney stones). Her calcium is elevated and her parathyroid hormone is within the normal range.
(5) A 45-year-old woman complains of more than 1 h of morning stiffness affecting both hands with subluxation of the metacarpal joints and inflammation of the proximal interphalangeal joints. She is anticitrullinated peptide antibody positive and her C-reactive protein is increased.

Question 22: MCQ

A 52-year-old woman has a neck lesion excised and is awaiting the pathology report. Which of the following would make this a neoplasia?

(a) Metastases identified in the lungs
(b) Local infiltration into neighbouring tissues
(c) Uncontrolled clonal expansion
(d) Non-caseating necrosis
(e) Identification of a genetic mutation

Question 23: True/False

There are vaccines available for a wide variety of microbes. Which of the following is true regarding vaccines?

(a) Dead vaccines, e.g. for influenza, induce humoral and cell-mediated immunity.
(b) The live vaccine is contraindicated in immunocompromised individuals.
(c) The measles, mumps and rubella vaccine increases the risk of autism.
(d) There is both a live attenuated and a killed vaccine for polio.
(e) A live attenuated vaccine may revert to its virulent form, causing disease.

Question 24: MCQ

A 25-year-old woman who uses tampons for menstruation presents with a fever, hypotension and diarrhoea and demonstrates an extensive blanching rash. She is managed appropriately and after 1 week there is desquamation including on the palms and soles. What is the most likely mechanism?

(a) Endotoxin-mediated activation of the complement pathway
(b) Drug hypersensitivity resulting in epidermal necrosis
(c) Shiga toxin cleavage of rRNA
(d) Non-specific binding of toxin to MHC II and T cell receptor
(e) Toxin-mediated ADP ribosylation of G-protein

Question 25: True/False

A 6-year-old boy immediately develops a widespread rash and facial swelling upon administration of IV amoxicillin. This describes a type I hypersensitivity reaction. Which of the following is true regarding hypersensitivity reactions?

(a) Free antigens cross-link IgM on sensitised basophils and mast cells, triggering degranulation in type I hypersensitivity.
(b) In type II hypersensitivity, antibodies bind to antigen, leading to lysis or phagocytosis.
(c) Rhesus disease of the newborn and hyperacute blood product transfusion reactions are examples of type III hypersensitivity reactions.
(d) A type IV hypersensitivity reaction, also known as delayed type hypersensitivity, is mediated by activated T cells.
(e) Type III reactions are caused by antigen–antibody complexes that are deposited on membranes and fix complement.

Question 26: MCQ

A 56-year-old man presents with back pain and weight loss, and is diagnosed with multiple myeloma. His laboratory tests demonstrate an M-protein spike on serum electrophoresis and impaired renal function, and echocardiography shows restrictive cardiomyopathy. On renal biopsy, which of the following may be present?

(a) Mesangial proliferation and IgA deposition
(b) Granulomatous inflammation and leukocytoplastic vasculitis
(c) Kimmelstiel–Wilson nodules
(d) Linear immunoglobulin deposition along basement membrane
(e) Apple green birefringence on Congo red staining

Question 27: SAQ (5 points)

One of the processes of cell injury is free radical induced. What are free radicals and what important reactions lead to cell injury?

Question 28: MCQ

A 45-year-old man presents with a 2-week history of low-grade fevers, malaise and fatigue. On examination, he is found to have a cardiac murmur and splinter haemorrhages. Echocardiography confirms subacute endocarditis. Which of the following is the most likely organism?

(a) *Streptococcus pyogenes*
(b) *Streptococcus sanguis*
(c) Enterococcus
(d) *Haemophilus aprophilus*
(e) *Eikenella corrodens*

Question 29: EMQ

A Anti-NAChR antibody
B Anti-double-stranded DNA antibody
C Anticentromere antibody
D Antimitochondrial antibody
E Anti-basement membrane antibody
F Anti-SSA antibody
G Antiendomysial antibody
H Antineutrophil cytoplasmic antibody
I Anti-smooth muscle antibody

For each of the scenarios below, choose the most appropriate antibody test from the list above.

(1) A 32-year-old woman presents with fatigue, facial rash over the cheeks, oral ulcers, joint pain, photosensitivity and past medical history of Reynaud's phenomenon.
(2) A 23-year-old woman presents with worsening tiredness and weakness as the day progresses with difficulty climbing stairs, swallowing difficulties, diplopia and ptosis.
(3) A 42 year old with a history of haemoptysis (blood-stained cough), haematuria and oronasal symptoms presents with an acutely red inflamed eye and renal failure.
(4) A 3 year old presents with chronic diarrhoea and difficulty gaining weight secondary to intolerance to gliadin. The small intestine demonstrates villous atrophy.
(5) A condition with intrahepatic biliary duct destruction resulting in biliary stasis and liver cirrhosis.

Question 30: EMQ

A Membranous glomerulonephritis
B Rapidly progressive glomerulonephritis

C Goodpasture syndrome
D Granulomatous polyangiitis (Wegener granulomatosis)
E Systemic lupus erythematosus
F Autosomal dominant polycystic kidney disease
G Autosomal recessive polycystic kidney disease
H Renal cell carcinoma
I Diabetic nephropathy
J Focal segmental glomerular sclerosis
K Minimal change disease
L Alport syndrome
M IgA nephropathy

For each of the scenarios below, choose the most appropriate answer from the list.

(1) A 3 month old presents with abdominal masses, urinary tract infection, haematuria and metabolic acidosis.

(2) A patient with haemoptysis and haematuria demonstrates a linear pattern on immunofluorescence of renal biopsy.

(3) Kimmelstiel–Wilson nodules are seen in a renal biopsy.

(4) A 4 year old presents with hypoalbuminaemia and oedema; the renal biopsy is normal on light microscopy but responds well to steroid therapy.

(5) A child with hearing and visual impairments whose mother also complains of haematuria.

Answers to Exam 1

Answer 1: MCQ
See *Pathology at a Glance* (**Disordered cell growth**).
(c) The normal histology of the distal oesophagus is stratified squamous epithelium. The biopsy demonstrated a change in the cell type to columnar epithelium. The process of change of cell type to another differentiated cell type is called metaplasia. In this case, this is due to chronic inflammation secondary to gastroesophageal reflux disease called Barrett oesophagus. It is believed to be associated with an increased risk of oesophageal adenocarcinoma.

Answer 2: MCQ
See *Pathology at a Glance* (**Atherosclerosis**).
(c) Sudden plaque rupture exposes the circulating platelets and coagulation factors to subendothelial collagen and thrombogenic components. This forms a thrombus, which if large enough will completely occlude the coronary vessel, leading to loss of distal blood supply. The cardiomyocytes will then undergo coagulation necrosis (d).

Answer 3: True/False
See *Pathology at a Glance* (**Cell death**).
(a) **False**
(b) **False**
(c) **True**
(d) **False**
(e) **True**

Even in the face of insults, cells can respond to repair and survive but certain changes indicate that cell death will occur: nuclear pyknosis (irreversible chromatin condensation), karyolysis (dissolution of chromatin matter) and karyorrhexis (irreversible nuclear fragmentation, lysosome rupture and autolysis, lysis of endoplasmic reticulum, vacuolisation of mitochondria).

Answer 4: SAQ
See *Pathology at a Glance* (**Thrombosis**).
The coagulation factors are typically proteases. Upon vascular damage factor VII comes into contact with tissue factor that produces an activated complex (TF-FVIIa) (1). This along with Ca^{2+} and a phospholipid surface activates factor IX and X (2). Factor Xa with factor Va, Ca^{2+} and phospholipid membrane activate prothrombin (II) to thrombin (IIa) (3). This activates fibrinogen (I) to fibrin (4) that is able to form a cross-linked clot with factor XIIIa (5).

Answer 5: MCQ
See *Pathology at a Glance* (**Infection and immunodeficiency**).
(d) Malaria is caused by intracellular parasites in the genus *Plasmodium*: *P. vivax*, *P. malariae*, *P. ovale*, *P. falciparum* and *P. knowlesi*. *Plasmodium vivax* is the most common cause of malaria worldwide, But *P. falciparum* causes the most severe infections. The transmission vector is the female *Anopheles* mosquito which ingests gametocytes from an infected animal, which undergo development into sporozoites that are then found in the mosquito saliva ready to infect another host. The sporozoites initially infect hepatocytes where they undergo multiplication and differentiation into merozoites. When ready, they will rupture the hepatocytes and then infect erythrocytes. In erythrocytes, the same cycle will occur whereby division and differentiation occur, and then cell rupture with infection of further erythrocytes. In the erythrocyte stage, some merozoites will differentiate into gametocytes that can be ingested by mosquitoes again.

Answer 6: EMQ
See *Pathology at a Glance* (**Disordered cell growth, and other chapters**).
(1) **F**. Patients with HIV/AIDS are increased risk of developing Kaposi sarcoma which is associated with HHV-8. In healthy individuals, the virus seems to be controlled by the immune system without any symptoms or signs but HIV patients are unable to mount a response.
(2) **E**. HPV 16, 18 and 31 are particularly associated with cervical epithelial infection and production of oncogenes. HPV is also associated with penile, anal and oropharyngeal carcinoma.
(3) **D**. Epstein–Barr virus is a double-stranded DNA virus that infects epithclial cells and B cells. Burkitt lymphoma remains a common malignancy in children in Africa although cases outside Africa also occur. The c-myc gene function is affected in Burkitt commonly due to the t8;14 translocation. The lymphoma is histologically characterised by sheets of lymphocytes with macrophages, giving the classic 'starry sky' appearance.
(4) **B**. The patient probably has hepatocellular carcinoma secondary to chronic hepatitis B virus infection. Hepatocellular carcinoma is also associated with hepatitis C, alcohol abuse and haemochromatosis but not hepatitis A infection (c).
(5) **D**. Previous EBV infection is linked to an increased risk of nasopharyngeal carcinoma and Burkitt lymphoma as well as post-transplant lymphoproliferative disorder.

Answer 7: MCQ
See *Pathology at a Glance* (**Tuberculosis**).
(b) Tuberculosis is caused by acid-fast bacilli, *Mycobacterium tuberculosis*. It is spread in air droplets and can be primary or secondary. In primary TB, a granuloma called a Ghon focus develops, usually with lymphadenopathy. This may progress to resolution and removal of the infection but alternatively the bacteria may remain in a dormant stage which can reactivate to form secondary infection at a later time. The other tests are appropriate for systemic lupus erythematosus (a), sarcoidosis (c) and amyloidosis (Congo red).

Answer 8: SAQ
See *Pathology at a Glance* (**Disordered cell growth**).
Hyperplasia – proliferation of cells; reversible; benign prostatic hyperplasia, endometrial hyperplasia

Dysplasia – growth of cells with abnormal size, shape, pigmentation and mitotic rate; reversible; cervical intraepithelial neoplasia

Anaplasia – abnormal reversal of differentiation of cells; irreversible; feature of many malignancies, e.g. Wilms' tumour

Neoplasia – excessive clonal proliferation of cells that is uncontrolled; irreversible; oesophageal adenocarcinoma

Hypertrophy – increase in cell size; reversible; cardiac hypertrophy secondary to hypertension, skeletal muscle hypertrophy with weight training

Answer 9: True/False
See *Pathology at a Glance* (Infection and immunodeficiency).
(a) **True**.
(b) **True**. This is achieved by reverse transcriptase packaged in the virus.
(c) **False**. Mother-to-child transmission can occur through all three mechanisms. The other modes of transmission are through blood products, sexual contact and needle sharing. Transmission risk is higher in male-to-male sexual intercourse compared to female-to-male and male-to-female transmission.
(d) **False**. Upon HIV transmission, an acute infection occurs, often with flu-like symptoms that may go unnoticed. This is followed by a latency period where the immune system response controls the viral load. After a variable period of time, usually years, the cell-mediated response is exhausted, with a drop in CD4 lymphocytes and antibodies and an increase in viral load. The patient is susceptible to a wide variety of opportunistic infections: AIDS.
(e) **True**. HAART remains the most effective treatment to control HIV/AIDS infections. Usually treatment is initiated with two nucleoside analogue reverse transcriptase inhibitors and one non-nucleoside analogue reverse transcriptase inhibitor or viral protease inhibitor. As new classes of drugs have been introduced, e.g. fusion inhibitors, integrase inhibitors, they have been integrated into treatment guidelines.

Answer 10: MCQ
See *Pathology at a Glance* (Acute inflammation).
(a) Neutrophils enter into sites of inflammation through a process involving rolling, tight binding, diapedesis and migration. Tight binding involves leucocyte integrin binding to ICAM-1 on vascular endothelium. This is followed by leucocyte passage between endothelial cells (diapedesis) and then migration guided by chemotactic agents such as cytokines. In sites of inflammation there is increased vsascular permeability and vasodilation mediated by, for example, histamine, bradykinin and complement.

Answer 11: MCQ
See *Pathology at a Glance* (Arthritis).
(a) Acute attacks of gout are caused by uric acid crystals deposited into joints causing an acute inflammatory reaction. Pseudogout is a similar condition caused by the deposition of calcium pyrophosphate crystals within the joint. On synovial fluid examination, there are rhomboid crystals that are weakly positively birefringent.

Answer 12: SAQ
See *Pathology at a Glance* (Infection and immunodeficiency).
Any five of the following.
  Faecal-oral: polio, hepatitis A, hepatitis E
  Sexual transmission: HIV, hepatitis B
  Blood products, contaminated IV needles: HIV, hepatitis B, hepatitis C

Respiratory droplets: influenza, measles, mumps, varicella zoster
  Sexual transmission: hepatitis B, IIIV
  Saliva: Epstein–Barr virus, herpes simplex virus
  Direct lesion contact: herpes simplex virus, varicella zoster
  Vectors: dengue (mosquitoes), West Nile virus (mosquitoes)
  Animal bite: rabies

Answer 13: MCQ
See *Pathology at a Glance* (Glomerulonephritis).
(c) Amyloid light chain (AL) amyloidosis is derived from immunoglobulin light chains produced in multiple myeloma. Amyloidosis can affect any organ but common problems include renal failure, restrictive cardiomyopathy, gastrointestinal, pulmonary and skin abnormalities. A second common cause of amyloidosis is AA amyloidosis caused by deposition of serum amyloid-associated protein, a condition seen in chronic inflammatory disease such as rheumatoid arthritis. Amyloid deposition is also seen in Alzheimer disease (β-amyloid), diabetes mellitus and medullary carcinoma of the thyroid.

Answer 14: EMQ
See *Pathology at a Glance* (Infection and immunodeficiency).
(1) **A**. A failure in the development of the third and fourth pharyngeal pouches causes thymic and parathyroid aplasia leading to recurrent infections and hypocalcaemia. Other features that may be present are abnormal facies, cleft palate, cardiac abnormalities (especially tetralogy of Fallot) and learning difficulties.
(2) **F**. Capsules are resistant to phagocytosis and therefore opsonins such as antibodies and complement are required. The spleen contains many macrophages for phagocytosis and removal of these pathogens. Other encapsulated bacteria include *Klebsiella pneumoniae*, *Salmonella typhi* and *Streptococcus agalactiae*.
(3) **D**. These patients are susuceptible to various opportunistic infections including Aspergillus, *Staphylococcus aureus*, Salmonella and *E. coli*. The nitroblue tetrazolium test is used to assess the activity of the enzyme. Reduction of nitroblue tetrazolium (i.e. normal function) gives a change in colour to blue.
(4) **B**. Bruton's agammaglobulinaemia is due to a tyrosine kinase defect affecting B cell production and therefore antibody responses. After maternal immunity is lost when breastfeeding stops, the infant becomes susceptible to recurrent infections.
(5) **C**. Phagocytes can be seen to have abnormal large lysosomes and recurrent infections. Also associated with peripheral neuropathy and oculocutaneous albinism.

Answer 15: MCQ
See *Pathology at a Glance* (Thrombosis).
(e) Virchow's triad comprises stasis, hypercoagulability and endothelial damage. Each of these is affected by a wide variety of factors, e.g. endothelial damage caused by hypertension, trauma, bacteria and inflammation. Deep vein thrombosis in this case is promoted by venous stasis. This thrombus is at risk of embolising to the pulmonary arteries, causing ventilation/perfusion mismatch.

Answer 16: SAQ

See *Pathology at a Glance* (**Ischemic heart disease, Myocardial and pericardial disease**).

Any five of the following.

Cardiac arrhythmia (½pt) – the infarcted tissue demonstrates different conduction properties to normal cardiac tissue, providing a substrate for potentially lethal ventricular fibrillation or tachycardia (½). Alternatively bradycardias may be seen if the electrical conduction pathway is damaged – most commonly seen with right coronary artery occlusion (½).

Acute pericarditis (½pt) – infarction leads to necrosis and inflammation which can extend into the pericardium (½). Note that acute pericarditis occurs within 1 week typically which is different from Dressler syndrome seen typically >2 weeks after the infarction.

Dressler syndrome (½pt) – autoimmune fibrinous pericarditis occurring typically >2 weeks after the infarction.

Ventricular free wall rupture (½pt) – occurring typically within 3–5 days of infarct as the myocardium undergoes necrosis, inflammation with infiltration of leucocytes and granulation tissue formation. The wall is left weakened and at risk of rupture (½). Leads to cardiac tamponade.

Papillary muscle rupture - as with ventricular free wall rupture.

Interventricular septal rupture – as with ventricular free wall rupture.

Cardiogenic shock (½pt) – reduced myocardial contractility secondary to loss of myocardium (½).

Ventricular aneurysm (½pt) – after the MI, the myocardium undergoes necrosis which is followed by inflammation and then replacement of normal tissue with scar tissue (½). A thrombus may form within an aneurysm due to blood stagnation.

Left ventricular thrombus (½pt) – a thrombus may form within an aneurysm due to blood stagnation secondary to a poorly mobile ventricular wall (½).

Answer 17: MCQ

See *Pathology at a Glance* (**Assorted haematological conditions**).

(e) Haemolytic-uraemic syndrome typically demonstrates thrombocytopenia (low platelets), microangiopathic haemolytic anaemia (MAHA) and acute kidney injury. The peripheral smear demonstrates schistocytes, which are fragments of erythrocytes and are classic for MAHA. Haemolytic-uraemic syndrome is classically preceded by diarrhea caused by *Escherichia coli* 0157:H7 or Shigella. Other important causes of MAHA include thrombotic thrombocytopenic purpura (TTP) and disseminated intravascular coagulation.

Answer 18: EMQ

See *Pathology at a Glance* (**Lymphoma, Oncogenes and tumour suppressor genes**).

(1) **E.** Chronic myelogenous leukaemia (CML), also called chronic myeloid leukaemia, is characterised by uncontrolled proliferation of granulocytes. It is characterised by the Philadelphia chromosome which is a translocation of chromosome 22 and 9 leading to fusion of the BCR and ABL genes. CML may accelerate to AML.

(2) **G.** Reed–Sternberg cells are necessary for a diagnosis of Hodgkin lymphoma but are also seen in other conditions, e.g. infectious mononucleosis. They are derived from B cells and are CD30 and CD15 positive. Hodgkin lymphoma can be associated with B-symptoms, i.e. fever, night sweats and weight loss. Epstein–Barr virus infection is associated with approximately half of all cases but do not confuse Burkitt lymphoma, a type of non-Hodgkin lymphoma.

(3) **F.** CLL is often incidentally diagnosed by physician examination or laboratory tests demonstrating very high white cell counts. However, it can present with non-specific symptoms such as fevers, sweats, weight loss and lethargy. The increased fragility of lymphocytes is seen as increased smudge cells. Note that CLL and small lymphocyte lymphoma (a B cell non-Hodgkin lymphoma) are considered the same spectrum of disease.

(4) **D.** AML is a rapidly progressing disease infiltrating the bone marrow with myeloblasts leading eventually to suppression of other cell lines including anaemia, thrombocytopenia (low platelets) and functional leucocytes. Auer rods are more commonly seen in the M3 or acute promyelocytic leukaemia type of AML, and are especially sensitive to all-trans retinoic acid. These patients are at high risk of disseminated intravascular coagulation (DIC).

(5) **I.** B cell leukaemia/lymphoma 2 (bcl-2) is an oncogene that prevents apoptosis upon activation. However, follicular lymphoma development requires other genetic events in addition to bcl-2 activation. Follocular lymphoma is one of the most common non-Hodgkin lymphomas and is characterised by small cleaved follicle cells and larger non-cleaved follicle cells.

Answer 19: MCQ

See *Pathology at a Glance* (**Body's natural defenses**).

(b) The question describes angio-oedema in the setting of minor trauma which is classic for hereditary angio-oedema caused by C1 esterase deficiency. The swelling is caused by bradykinin. C2 and C4 will be low if measured.

Answer 20: MCQ

See *Pathology at a Glance* (**Alcoholic and non-alcoholic liver disease**).

(c) Mallory bodies, named after American pathologist Frank Mallory, are classic in alcoholic hepatitis. These are inclusions within hepatocytes of 'rope-like' tangled cytokeratin and other proteins which are eosinophilic on H&E staining. The presence of fibrosis indicates repeated injury to the liver.

Answer 21: EMQ

See *Pathology at a Glance* (**Miscellaneous non-neoplastic osteoarticular pathology**).

(1) **E.** A newly inflamed tender joint is most probably associated with septic arthritis, pseudogout or gout. The demonstration of needle-shaped crystals that are negatively birefringent is typical of the uric acid crystals seen in gout. Rhomboid positively birefringent crystals are seen in pseudogout (d). Septic arthritis must always be ruled out in an acutely inflamed joint. *Staphylococcus aureus* is the most common cause, but *Neisseria gonorrhoeae* is common in young, sexually active adults and Salmonella is common in sickle cell patients. Other gram-negative organisms may also be involved.

(2) **F.** Osteoporosis is a decrease in bone mineral density predisposing to fractures. Risk factors include increasing age, female gender, steroid use and hypogonadism.

(3) **A.** The radiographic findings are classic for osteoarthritis. Subchondral sclerosis is another finding that may be described. A history of trauma to the joint predisposes to osteoarthritis.

(4) **I.** Although the parathyroid hormone is within the normal range, in a hypercalcaemic patient the parathyroid hormone is suppressed. Parathyroid adenoma and hyperplasia are the most common causes of primary hyperparathyroidism. In these patients you may also see hypophosphataemia (as PTH increases renal phosphate loss) and increased 1,25-dihydroxycholecalciferol (calcitriol).

(5) **B.** Rheumatoid arthritis is an inflammatory, destructive, symmetrical polyarthropathy of unknown cause. Morning stiffness and bilateral hand involvement are common, and a positive anti-CCP is highly specific for the disease.

Answer 22: MCQ

See *Pathology at a Glance* (**Disordered cell growth, Basic concepts in neoplasia**).

(c) Neoplasia is defined by an uncontrolled proliferation of cells, and they may be benign or cancerous. Metastases (spread to a non-adjacent tissue) is a feature of a malignant neoplasm but is also seen in infections (a). Similarly, (b) is also a feature of malignant tumours. Necrosis may be seen in both benign (e.g. due to pressure) or malignant neoplasms, as well as a wide variety of other processes (e).

Answer 23: True/False

See *Pathology at a Glance* (**Inflammation and immunity**).

(a) **False.** Live attenuated vaccines induce both humoral and cell-mediated immunity but killed vaccines only induce a humoral response.

(b) **True.** Due to the risk of developing a dangerous infection in immunocompromised individuals. Live vaccines include MMR, Sabin polio, varicella zoster and smallpox.

(c) **False.** A scare was created by a famous paper (later proven to be seriously flawed) which suggested that the MMR vaccine increases the risk of autism. Further studies have shown no such association.

(d) **True.** The Salk killed virus was developed first and then subsequently the Sabin live attenuated virus was produced.

(e) **True.** This is rare but has been demonstrated to occur, for example Sabin polio vaccination.

Answer 24: MCQ

See *Pathology at a Glance*.

(d) The clue is the use of a tampon which is classically associated with toxic shock syndrome (TSS). TSS is caused by the *Staphylococcus aureus* toxin which acts as a superantigen to bind to MHC II and non-specifically activates large numbers of T cells. The subsequent cytokine milieu causes a severe, potentially fatal condition. A similar condition not associated with tampon use can be caused by toxin released by *Streptococcus pyogenes*.

Answer 25: True/False

See *Pathology at a Glance* (**Hypersensitivity reactions**).

(a) **False.** IgE are cross-linked to cause degranulation and release of cytokines and inflammatory mediators, e.g. histamine. These cells also produce a secondary set of mediators from arachidonic acid that are important for the slower prolonged inflammation, e.g. leukotrienes.

(b) **True.** Complement activation leads to formation of the membrane attack complex which forms pores in the target cell and cell lysis. Both antibodies and complement may act as opsonins for phagocytosis.

(c) **False.** Rhesus disease of the newborn occurs due to maternally derived antibodies against the Rhesus antigen on erythrocytes. Hyperacute blood transfusion reactions occur due to preformed antibodies. Both lead to destruction of erythrocytes which are targeted and destroyed. Therefore, it is a type II reaction. Other examples include myasthenia gravis, Graves' disease, Goodpasture syndrome and bullous pemphigoid.

(d) **True.** Type IV hypersensitivity reactions are not antibody dependent unlike types I–III. They require antigen-presenting cells activating presensitised T cells to release cytokines, and activate macrophages and cytotoxic T cells.

(e) **True.** Type III hypersensitivity reactions include Arthus reaction (local reaction to an intradermal antigen injection), systemic lupus erythematosus, rheumatoid arthritis and poststreptococcal glomerulonephritis.

Answer 26: MCQ

See *Pathology at a Glance* (**Myeloma**).

(e) Apple green birefringence of Congo red-stained preparation under polarised light microscopy is classic for amyloidosis. It is caused by immunoglobulin light chains in multiple myeloma. It also explains this patient's restrictive cardiomyopathy. Amyloidosis of different organs is seen in a variety of conditions including chronic inflammatory conditions (AA amyloidosis), Alzheimer disease, haemodialysis associated (β2-microglobulin), diabetes mellitus. (a) describes IgA nephropathy, (b) granulomatous poly-angiitis (previously called Wegener granulomatosis), (c) describes diabetic nephropathy, (d) describes Goodpasture syndrome.

Answer 27: SAQ

See *Pathology at a Glance* (**Tissue damage**).

Free radicals are species with a single unpaired electron in their outer shell (1). They are extremely reactive and unstable chemicals that damage nucleic acids and organelle membrane (2). DNA fragmentation secondary to single-strand breaks due to reactions with thymine in nucleic acids (3). Protein cross-linking affecting function (including enzymes) (4). Free radical attack of membrane polyunsaturated lipids yielding unstable peroxides (5). Free radical reaction leading to polypeptide fragmentation (6).

Answer 28: MCQ

See *Pathology at a Glance* (**Cardiac valvular disease**).

(b) Endocarditis is an inflammation of the endocardium, the inner lining of the heart, and typically involves the cardiac valves. *Streptococcus sanguis* is a viridans group streptococcus, which are the most common cause of subacute endocarditis. The other bacteria are less common causes of endocarditis. (d) and (e) are among the HACEK organisms (fastidious gram-negative bacilli: *Haemophilus aphrophilus*, *Actinobacillus actinomycetem-comitans*, *Cardiobacterium hominis*, *Eikenella corrodens* and *Kingella kingae*). *Staphylococcus aureus* is commonly seen in rapidly progressing endocarditis often associated with intravenous drug use.

Answer 29: EMQ

See *Pathology at a Glance* (Systemic vasculitis).

(1) **B**. The vignette describes systemic lupus erythematosus which is more common in females and has widespread effects. The most sensitive antibody is antinuclear antibody, which is very non-specific. Anti-ds DNA and anti-Smith antibodies are both more specific for SLE. Drug-induced SLE, e.g. due to hydralazine, isoniazid, may have antihistone antibodies.

(2) **A**. Myasthenia gravis is a disorder of the neuromuscular junction that more commonly affects young women. Management involves symptomatic treatment with acetylcholinesterase inhibitors and immunosuppressive treatment, e.g. steroids and azathioprine.

(3) **H**. Of the autoimmune conditions, Goodpasture syndrome and Wegener granulomatosis (recently renamed granulomatosis polyangiitis) both affect the lungs and kidneys. They can both cause rapidly progressive glomerulonephritis. However, Wegener is more commonly associated with widespread systemic effects. ANCA can be of two forms: cANCA is particularly associated with Wegener whereas p-ANCA is less specific and may be associated with, for example, microscopic polyangiitis and Churg–Strauss syndrome.

(4) **G**. Coeliac disease can present in any age group and is a common cause of malabsorption. Both antiendomysial and anti-tissue transglutaminase antibodies are associated with this condition. Treatment is a gluten-free diet.

(5) **D**. Describes primary biliary cirrhosis.

Answer 30: EMQ

See *Pathology at a Glance* (Glomerulonephritis, **Important types of glomerulonephritis**).

(1) **G**. Autosomal recessive polycystic kidney disease is significantly less common than the adult variant (f) and is associated with hepatic cysts. The disease is associated with PKHD1 mutation. It typically results in end-stage renal failure within the first two decades of life and also a decline in liver function. Pulmonary hypoplasia is a common consequence of the polycystic kidneys.

(2) **C**. Although haemoptysis and haematuria may be seen in both (c) and (d), the immunofluorescence pattern is typical of Goodpasture syndrome with antiglomerular basement membrane. The disease can be rapidly progressing.

(3) **I**. In diabetes mellitus, the first change is glomerular basement membrane thickening leading to mesangial expansion. As the disease worsens, progressive nodular glomerulosclerosis (Kimmelstiel–Wilson nodules) destroy the nephrons. As this expands renal function continues to worsen.

(4) **K**. Hypoalbuminaemia, massive proteinuria (>3.5 g per day) and oedema is the triad of nephrotic syndrome. It is the most common cause of nephrotic syndrome in childhood. Electron microscopy would have demonstrated podocyte foot process effacement.

(5) **L**. The condition described is Alport syndrome associated with type IV collagen defect. It presents as a nephritic syndrome and can progress to end-stage renal failure. Sensorineural hearing loss and visual impairment due to a wide variety of ocular disorders are commonly associated.

10 Pathology exam 2

Questions

Question 1: EMQ
A Pancreatic adenocarcinoma
B Cholelithiasis
C Cholangitis
D Primary sclerosing cholangitis
E Primary biliary cirrhosis
F Pancreatic necrosis
G Gilbert syndrome
H Dubin–Johnson syndrome
I Hepatocellular carcinoma
J None of the above

For each of the following scenarios choose the most appropriate answers from the list above.
(1) A 42-year-old overweight woman presents with right upper quadrant abdominal pain, fever and jaundice. She reports a history of similar pain after meals for the past 4–5 months.
(2) A 54 year old presents with progressively worsening jaundice, weight loss and a palpable gallbladder without pain.
(3) A 34-year-old man with a long history of ulcerative colitis presents with jaundice. On ERCP there is intrahepatic and extrahepatic biliary tree strictures and dilation.
(4) A 34 year old with a urinary tract infection is found to have mildly raised unconjugated bilirubin. Retesting of liver functions after 1 month demonstrates resolution. A few years later when she is admitted for pneumonia, the bilirubin is again mildly raised.
(5) A 43 year old with systemic lupus erythematosus presents with jaundice. Blood tests demonstrate a raised unconjugated bilirubin and raised reticulocyte count.

Question 2: MCQ
A 34-year-old man is involved in a road traffic accident with significant haemorrhage. He is known to be O Rh+. Which blood group can he receive?
(a) A Rh-
(b) AB Rh+
(c) AB Rh-
(d) B Rh-
(e) All of the above
(f) None of the above

Question 3: EMQ
A Folic acid
B Thiamine
C Vitamin B$_{12}$
D Retinol
E Vitamin C
F Vitamin D
G Biotin
H Niacin
I Vitamin K

For each of the scenarios below choose the most appropriate answer from the list above.
(1) A 43-year-old alcoholic who presents with ophthalmoplegia, gait ataxia and confusion. Which deficiency is the likely cause?
(2) A 12-year-old recent immigrant from India presents with poor wound healing, gum bleeding, ecchymoses (bruising) and coiled hairs. Which deficiency is the likely cause?
(3) A 53-year-old man who is currently being treated for tuberculosis presents with diarrhoea, widespread hyperpigmented rash, disorientation and confusion. Which deficiency is the likely cause?
(4) A 22 year old with cystic fibrosis presents with easy bruisability, gum bleeding and haematuria due to a failure in γ-carboxylation. Which deficiency is the likely cause?
(5) A medical student on a visit to a village in Uganda meets a young boy with measles. A few weeks ago he complains of poor vision at night. Which mineral should be administered?

Question 4: MCQ
A 50-year-old man dies in a motor vehicle accident. The cross-section of his heart from the autopsy is shown in Figure 10.1. What condition did he probably have?

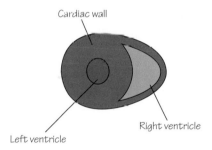

Figure 10.1 Schematic transverse section of the patient's heart following autopsy.

(a) Amyloidosis
(b) Alcoholism
(c) Sarcoidosis
(d) Hypertension
(e) Pericarditis

Question 5: EMQ
A *Clostridium difficile*
B *Clostridium botulinum*
C *Streptococcus agalactiae*
D *Neisseria meningitides*
E Shigella
F *Helicobacter pylori*
G *Bartonella henselae*

H *Leptospira interrogans*
I *Borrelia burgdorferi*
J *Chlamydia trachomatis*

For each of the questions below, choose the most appropriate micro-organism from the list above.

(1) A 42 year old has returned from a camping trip. He reports being bitten many times by insects. He presents now with a facial nerve palsy but reports having had a rash preceding this. What is the infecting organism?

(2) A 34 year old presents with severe abdominal pain for the past 3–4 weeks that is worse on eating meals. His condition is associated with a gram-negative rod that produces urease. What is the causative organism?

(3) A 3 year old presents with complete paralysis soon after lunch caused by a toxin that inhibits acetylcholine release at the neuromuscular junction by acting on SNARE proteins.

(4) A 12 year old presents with fevers and a widespread purpuric rash caused by gram-negative cocci with a polysaccharide capsule.

(5) A major cause of neonatal septicaemia which can be found in the vagina.

Question 6: MCQ

A 4-year-old girl on routine physical examination is found to have a left abdominal mass. An 8 cm renal mass is resected and histology of the mass demonstrates primitive tubules with immature spindle cells. There are no metastases. What is the most likely diagnosis?

(a) Wilms tumour
(b) Renal medullary carcinoma
(c) Renal cell carcinoma
(d) Neuroblastoma
(e) Phaeochromocytoma

Question 7: True/False

One of the components of the innate immune system is the complement system which requires hepatic proteins C1 to C9. Which of the following is true regarding the complement cascade?

(a) C3b acts as an opsonin by binding to antigens and enhancing phagocytosis.
(b) C1 inhibitor acts as a chemotactic agent towards neutrophils and monocytes.
(c) C3a nd C5a induce mast cell degranulation and cause increased vascular permeability.
(d) C1–C5 form the membrane attack complex that forms pores on target cells.
(e) Regulation of the complement pathway is impaired in C1 inhibitor deficiency, leading to spontaneous angio-oedema.

Question 8: SAQ (5 points)

Down syndrome is a trisomy disorder characterised by multiple abnormalities. Name the trisomy (1 point) and the two most common mechanisms by which the trisomy occurs (2 points). Name two other trisomies that survive to birth (2 points).

Question 9: MCQ

A 42-year-old woman presents with right back pain and discomfort on urination. She has a known history of multiple urinary tract infections. On urinalysis, pH 7.5 and crystals are found. On CT scan, she is found to have a right staghorn renal calculus. What is the most likely composition of the crystals?

(a) Calcium oxalate
(b) Magnesium ammonium phosphate
(c) Uric acid
(d) Cystine
(e) Calcium phosphate

Question 10: True/False

A 27-year-old pregnant woman undergoes an ultrasound that leads to a diagnosis of hydatiform mole. Which of the following is true?

(a) A complete mole has only a maternal origin with no paternal DNA.
(b) Fetal parts are seen in complete moles.
(c) One of the complications of a molar pregnancy is the development of choriocarcinoma.
(d) β-Human chorionic gonadotropin rise after removal of a molar pregnancy may indicate malignancy.
(e) Excess β-hCG can lead to hyperthyroidism.

Question 11: MCQ

A 14-year-old boy presents to the emergency department with chest pain and shortness of breath. His chest X-ray shows infiltration, his peripheral blood smear shows sickle cells and his Hb is 6.5 g/dL. Which of the following describes the underlying pathology?

(a) Point mutation of β-globin at position 6
(b) Deletion in α-globin gene
(c) Reduced production of β-globins
(d) Mutation of spectrin or ankyrin gene
(e) None of the above

Question 12: SAQ (5 points)

A 42-year-old woman presents with a lump in the left breast. List five risk factors for breast malignancy (2.5 points). Which of the following are malignant or benign: fibroadenoma, intraductal papilloma, Paget disease of the breast, fat necrosis and ductal carcinoma?

Question 13: MCQ

A 34-year-old Indian man is diagnosed with tuberculosis. All of the following regarding tuberculosis are true except:

(a) It requires prolonged treatment with multiple drugs.
(b) It can cause spinal infection.
(c) Detection requires acid-fast staining.
(d) Patients infected with *M. tuberculosis* are almost always symptomatic.
(e) BCG vaccine is the only one available.

Question 14: True/False

The immune system can be divided into innate and adaptive. The latter provides a prolonged, stronger pathway that can demonstrate memory. Which of the following is true regarding lymphocytes?

(a) Pathogens are phagocytosed by antigen-presenting cells (APCs) and processes for presentation.
(b) The first step in activation requires foreign antigen presentation on MHC I to CD4 T cells.
(c) Anergy results if the CD4 T cell does not receive a second signal.

(d) B cells are APCs that require CD4 T cell activation before antigen presentation.

(e) CD8 T cells recognise antigens presented by APCs as well as other cells.

Question 15: MCQ

A 62-year-old man with a 40 pack-year smoking history presents with a bloody cough, weight loss and bone pain. His laboratory tests demonstrats a hypercalcaemia and low parathyroid hormone. Which of the following is most probably also present?

(a) A pleural malignancy
(b) Highly concentrated urine
(c) Additional symptoms of flushing, diarrhoea, wheezing and right-sided cardiac murmurs
(d) Cushingoid features with high ACTH
(e) A large hilar mass arising from the bronchus

Question 16: True/False

A 45-year-old man presents with abdominal pain after returning from a trip to Egypt 2 days ago. He has recently had unprotected sex. His laboratory tests demonstrate hepatitis A IgG positive, hepatitis B surface antigen negative, hepatitis B surface antibody positive, hepatitis B core antibody positive, hepatitis C antibody positive. Of note, he had a blood transfusion 16 years ago.

(a) The chronic hepatitis A infection was probably transmitted during the blood transfusion.
(b) Hepatitis B vaccination resulted in the antibody response for this patient.
(c) Co-infection with hepatitis D worsens hepatitis B infection prognosis.
(d) The window period refers to the period of hepatitis B where no surface antigen is present and surface antibody has not been produced.
(e) The presence of hepatitis B e antigen would indicate enhanced infectivity and high viral replication.

Question 17: MCQ

A 45-year-old man presents with acute kidney failure. Which of the following is most likely to be present?

(a) Hyperkalaemia
(b) Metabolic alkalosis
(c) Raised pCO_2
(d) Normal urea and creatinine
(e) All of the above

Question 18: True/False

A 42 year old who is being investigated for macrocytic anaemia is found to have hypersegmented neutrophils and megaloblasts. Which of the following is true?

(a) The causes of megaloblastic anaemia are cobalamin, folic acid and biotin deficiency.
(b) Vitamin B_{12} is a co-factor for homocysteine methyltransferase and methylmalonyl-CoA mutase.
(c) Terminal ileum inflammation in Crohn disease predisposes particularly to folate deficiency.
(d) Folic acid deficiency is associated with optic atrophy, dementia and subacute combined degeneration of the cord.
(e) Folic acid deficiency in pregnancy predisposes to neural tube defects.

Question 19: MCQ

A 54 year old presents with severe abdominal pain and on investigation is found to have significantly raised amylase and lipase with deranged liver function tests. Which of the following is the most common cause of the underlying disease?

(a) Gallstones
(b) Mumps
(c) Steroids
(d) Hypercalcaemia
(e) Thiazide diuretics

Question 20: MCQ

A 43-year-old woman on a regular primary care visit finds out she is pregnant. Which of the following drugs she uses is most likely to be teratogenic?

(a) Low molecular weight heparin
(b) Ibuprofen
(c) Alcohol
(d) Amoxicillin
(e) Paracetamol

Question 21: SAQ (5 points)

Congenital cardiac disease may present with cyanosis very early or later in childhood. Discuss three shunts found in the fetus and describe two congenital cardiac defects that lead to right-to-left shunting.

Question 22: MCQ

A 2 year old has dextrocardia, situs inversus, recurrent respiratory tract infections, bronchiectasis and infertility. Which of the following is the underlying cause?

(a) Defect in cilia motility
(b) Microtubule polymerisation defect
(c) Erythrocyte membrane protein mutation
(d) Lecithin deficiency
(e) Impaired chloride transporter

Question 23: SAQ (5 points)

A 45-year-old man develops renal failure secondary to diabetic nephropathy. He also develops calcitriol deficiency. Explain the cause and subsequent changes including calcium and phosphate levels, and to the bone.

Question 24: EMQ

A Berry aneurysms
B Raised LDL cholesterol
C Café-au-lait spots
D Trinucleotide repeat in Huntingtin gene
E Increased colonic polyps
F Increased risk of ovarian malignancy
G Aortic dissection
H Cardiomyopathy
I Trisomy 13

For each of the following, choose the most appropriate association from the list above.

(1) An 18 year old presents to the emergency department and is diagnosed with a myocardial infarction. He has a strong family history of early-onset cardiovascular disease. On examination he has tendon xanthoma.

(2) A tall 32-year-old man with long, thin digits and lens subluxation up and out (superotemporal). He has an underlying fibrillin gene mutation.

(3) Autosomal dominant disorder characterised with multiple neurofibromas and the presence of iris hamartomas. The patient also has a family history of phaeochromocytoma.

(4) A 32-year-old woman presents with abnormal limb movements, low mood and progressive dementia. An autopsy of her father demonstrated caudate atrophy.

(5) A 34 year old diagnosed with hypertension and renal failure secondary to polycystic kidney disease.

Question 25: MCQ

A 23 year old presents with multiple gastric ulcers and is diagnosed with multiple endocrine neoplasia. Which of the following neoplasms are associated with the condition?

(a) Parathyroid and phaechromocytoma
(b) Parathyroid and pituitary
(c) Neurofibroma and phaeochromocytoma
(d) Medullary thyroid carcinoma and pituitary
(e) Follicular thyroid and pituitary

Question 26: SAQ (5 points)

A 24-year-old man presents with haematochezia (bright red blood per rectum) and a several-month history of diarrhoea and weight loss. He is diagnosed with inflammatory bowel disease. List five comparisons between Crohn disease and ulcerative colitis.

Question 27: MCQ

A 62-year-old woman presents with intense headache and jaw pain on chewing. On examination, she has tenderness of the right temple and a biopsy of the artery demonstrates granulomatous inflammation. Which of the following is an associated condition?

(a) Ulcerative colitis
(b) Polymyalgia rheumatica
(c) Fibromyalgia
(d) Smoking
(e) Coronary artery aneurysms
(f) Psoriasis

Question 28: MCQ

A 34-year-old sexually active woman presents with a painless ulcer on the genitalia. She tests positive for VDRL. Which of the following is associated with causative infection?

(a) Hepatocellular carcinoma
(b) Fetal abnormalities
(c) Gram-positive on staining
(d) Hilar lymphadenopathy
(e) Pustular penile discharge

Question 29: True/False

A man is brought into hospital with breathing difficulty and is found to have infiltrates consistent with pneumonia. For each of the following choose true or false.

(a) Gram-positive diplococcus is the most likely cause of a left lower lobe pneumonia.
(b) Cystic fibrosis patients are at increased risk of *Pseudomonas aeruginosa* pneumonia.
(c) Bilateral infiltrates, dry cough and desaturation on ambulation in a patient with a CD4 count of 150 cells/mm^3 are concerning for *Staphylococcus aureus*.
(d) Treatment with azithromycin will cover *Legionella pneumophila*.
(e) A several-week history with upper lobe involvement and microscopy would demonstrate caseating granulomas in mycoplasma infection.

Question 30: MCQ

During a routine examination, a 2 year old is found to have an abdominal mass. On biopsy, there are small round blue cells arising separate from the kidney. Which of the following is the likely neoplasm?

(a) Neuroblastoma
(b) Nephroblastoma (Wilms tumour)
(c) Retinoblastoma
(d) Hodgkin lymphoma
(e) Ewing sarcoma

Answers to Exam 2

Answer 1: EMQ
See *Pathology at a Glance* **(Hepatic and pancreaticobiliary disease)**.

(1) **C.** Risk factors for gallstone disease are 'female, forty, fatty and fertile'. Charcot's triad of right upper quadrant abdominal pain, fever and jaundice defines ascending cholangitis and if shock and mental status changes are present then it is Reynold's triad. Ascending cholangitis is an infection of the bile duct typically caused by an obstructive gallstone.

(2) **A.** Pancreatic adenocarcinoma of the head can create an obstructive jaundice. It has very poor prognosis as it metastasises early. CA-19-9 is used as a tumour marker. Courvoisier's sign refers to jaundice with a distended painless gallbladder.

(3) **D.** Primary sclerosing cholangitis is classically associated with ulcerative colitis. It is also more common in Crohn disease. It is characterised by intra- and extrahepatic inflammation and fibrosis of the biliary system. ERCP gives a classic 'beading' pattern due to the strictures and dilation.

(4) **G.** Gilbert syndrome is a benign congenital disorder associated with elevated unconjugated bilirubin at the time of stress such as an infection. The disease is caused by reduction in activity of glucuronyl transferase. Crigler–Najjar syndrome is associated with absence of this enzyme; it presents with jaundice and is fatal within the first few years of life. Dubin–Johnson syndrome (h) is due to a defect in excretion of bilirubin glucuronide. Rotor syndrome is within the spectrum of disease.

(5) **J.** The presence of raised unconjugated bilirubin is seen in Gilbert syndrome (G) as well as in haemolysis. Increased reticulocyte count suggests an increased cell turnover secondary to, in this case, haemolysis. Systemic lupus erythematosus is associated with warm autoimmune haemolytic anaemia and a direct Coombs test in this case would be positive.

Answer 2: MCQ
See *Pathology at a Glance* **(Assorted haematological conditions)**.

(e) The blood group is defined by the presence of surface antigens on erythrocytes. There are 30 blood group systems but the two most important ones are ABO and Rh. The ABO blood group system is determined by the presence of carbohydrate antigens on the erythrocytes. In blood type A, the A antigen is on the erythrocyte and the plasma will have anti-B antibodies; in blood type B, the B antigen is on the erythrocyte and the plasma will have anti-A antibodies; in blood type AB, both A and B antigens are present and no antibodies; and in blood type O, neither A or B antigens are present and both anti-A and anti-B antibodies appear in the plasma. Therefore, individuals who are blood type O cannot receive any other blood group except O, whereas AB individuals can receive any blood group.

In the Rh system, Rh- individuals can only receive Rh- blood whereas Rh+ can accept Rh- or Rh+ blood. The Rh- system is also important in Rh- mothers who are pregnant with Rh+ fetuses. This results in a haemolytic disease of the fetus due to IgG antibodies produced by the mother.

Answer 3: EMQ
See *Pathology at a Glance*.

(1) **B.** Wernicke encephalopathy is an acute neurological condition associated with thiamine deficiency commonly seen in alcoholics. Failure to treat Wernicke can lead to irreversible Korsakoff syndrome (KS). KS is associated with anterograde and retrograde amnesia and confabulation. Wernicke in alcoholics can especially be triggered by the administration of glucose before thiamine replacement. Wernicke encephalopathy is associated with lesions of the mammillary bodies, medial thalamus, third and fourth ventricles.

(2) **E.** Vitamin C (ascorbic acid) is essential for hydroxylation of proline and lysine amino acids in collagen synthesis. It is also important as a co-factor of several other enzymes including for norepinephrine synthesis from dopamine. Ascorbic acid is found in citrus fruits, tomatoes, cauliflowers, etc.

(3) **H.** Vitamin B_3 (niacin) is synthesised from trytophan and requires pyridoxine (vitamin B_6). Isoniazid, used in tuberculosis treatment, affects vitamin B_6 metabolism. Other causes of vitamin B_3 deficiency include carcinoid syndrome which increases tryptophan metabolism to produce serotonin, Hartnup disease (congenital disorder affecting tryptophan absorption) and other drugs, e.g. azathioprine, phenobarbital.

(4) **I.** Vitamin K is synthesised by gut flora and found in green vegetables. It is used by the body for γ-carboxylation of II, VII, IX, X, protein C and S. Therefore, patients have abnormal clotting and a bleeding disorder. The condition is also seen in neonates (lacking intestinal flora) and vitamin K treatment is often given in newborns.

(5) **D.** This question requires you to know that retinol is vitamin A which is required for the production of visual pigments in the eye. Deficiency is one of the most common causes of blindness in the developing world. Also, studies have shown that vitamin A administration in measles in the developing world reduces morbidity and mortality, and therefore should be part of routine treatment. The mechanism remains unknown.

Answer 4: MCQ
See *Pathology at a Glance* **(Systemic hypertension)**.

(d) The cross-section demonstrates a thickened left ventricle consistent with concentric hypertrophy seen in untreated hypertension. Alcoholism characteristically causes dilated cardiomyopathy whereas sarcoidosis and amyloidosis cause restrictive cardiomyopathy.

Answer 5: EMQ
See *Pathology at a Glance*.

(1) **I.** The presentation is classic for Lyme disease. It is caused by the spirochaete *Borrelia burgdorferi*, which is transmitted by the Ixodes tick (an ectoparasite). The classic rash, called erythema chronicum migrans, produces a 'bulls-eye' appearance. The disease can progress to cause acute neurological manifestations but also affects the heart (most commonly as atrioventricular block) and causes meningoencephalitis and arthritis.

(2) **F.** *Helicobacter pylori* is a gram-negative organism that is involved in peptic ulcers, and is a risk factor for gastric adenocarcinoma. It produces urease that breaks down urea to carbon dioxide and ammonia. Ammonia is converted to ammonium by accepting a proton, thereby creating an alkaline environment.

(3) **B.** *Clostridium perfringens* produces toxin that causes the paralysis. Death can occur due to respiratory failure. Clostridia are spore-forming anaerobic bacteria and also include *Clostridium tetani* (tetanus) and *Clostridium difficile* (pseudomembranous colitis).

(4) **D.** *Neisseria meningitidis*, along with streptococcus pneumonia and *Haemophilus influenzae*, is a major cause of meningitis, although vaccinations are now available against the three. In addition, in neonates, the immunocompromised and elderly, *Listeria monocytogenes* is another major cause. *N. meningitidis* is often part of the normal flora in the pharynx. It can cause a widespread septicaemia classically with purpuric rash without meningitis.

(5) **C.** *Streptococcus agalactiae* is a β-haemolytic gram-positive that is usually tested for in pregnant women as it can be a major cause of morbidity and mortality in the newborn, causing pneumonia, meningitis and septicaemia.

Answer 6: MCQ

See *Pathology at a Glance* (**Renal neoplasms**).

(a) The most common renal tumour in children is a nephroblastoma or Wilms tumour (named after the German surgeon who first described it). They can be associated with congenital syndromes including WAGR (Wilms tumour, aniridia, genitourinary abnormalities and mental retardation) and Denys–Drash syndrome. The case described here is classic. Histologically the tumour falls among neoplasms that show small blue round cells. Others include neuroblastoma, Ewing sarcoma and medulloblastoma.

Answer 7: True/False

See *Pathology at a Glance* (**The body's natural defences**).

(a) **True.** Neutrophils and macrophages (phagocytes) contain C3b receptors.

(b) **False.** C5a stimulates leucocyte activation and increases adhesion to the endothelium by integrins. It is also a chemotactic agent for various leucocytes.

(c) **True.**

(d) **False.** C5–C9 form these pores in microbes upon activation of the complement pathways. Deficiency in formation of the MAC predisposes to infections, especially *Neisseria*.

(e) **True.** Lack of downregulation of the complement pathway leads to excessive activation which leads to vasodilation and increased vascular permeability. The swelling can affect the face and airways, which is potentially life-threatening in hereditary angio-oedema.

Answer 8: SAQ

See *Pathology at a Glance* (**Genetic disease**).

Trisomies are typically fatal *in utero*. The three major trisomies that survive are 21 (Down), 18 (Edward) and 13 (Patau syndrome). However, the last two typically die during infancy. The most common cause of Down syndrome is meiotic non-disjunction, which refers to the failure of a chromosome pair to separate during

anaphase in meiosis 1 or meiosis 2. A less common cause is Robertsonian translocation where there is translocation of the long arm of chromosome 21 and chromosome 14.

Answer 9: MCQ

See *Pathology at a Glance*.

(b) Recurrent urinary tract infections caused by urea-splitting bacteria such as proteus result in increased ammonia production and urinary alkalinisation, leading to decreased phosphate solubility. Large calculi such as a staghorn may form. However, in the general population the most common cause of a urinary tract calculus is calcium-containing stones and in particular calcium oxalate (a). Cystine stones are rare and are associated with congenital defects in renal cystine handling (d).

Answer 10: True/False

See *Pathology at a Glance* (**Obstetric pathology**).

(a) **False.** A complete mole is produced from an ovum without DNA being fertilised by one sperm which undergoes mitosis or two sperms fertilising the egg. The genotype is most commonly 46XX. Findings of a molar pregnancy include large for gestational age uterus, hyperemesis gravidarum, early-onset pre-eclampsia, 'bunch of grapes' appearance on ultrasound and vaginal bleeding.

(b) **False.** Fetal parts may be present in partial moles which are derived from an egg fertilised by a sperm undergoing mitosis or by two sperm. The genotype is commonly triploid or tetraploid.

(c) **True.** Choriocarcinomas are trophoblastic malignant neoplasms, and can also be derived from ectopic, aborted or normal pregnancies.

(d) **True.** After removal of a complete or partial molar pregnancy, the β-hCG is typically monitored. A failure of disappearance or an increase in β-hCG can indicate the development of choriocarcinoma.

(e) **True.** This is a possible complication of choriocarcinomas which are associated with very high β-hCG levels that can stimulate the TSH receptor and therefore thyroid hormone production.

Answer 11: MCQ

See *Pathology at a Glance* (**Assorted haematological conditions**).

(a) Sickle cell anaemia is an autosomal recessive disorder caused by point mutations at chromosome 11 position 6 of the β-globin gene causing a change in amino acid from glutamine to valine. (b) and (c) describe causes of α- and β-thalassaemia. (d) describes causes of hereditary spherocytosis – other causes include band 3 protein and protein 4.2. All of these are important for maintaining the erythrocyte membrane and therefore shape.

Answer 12: SAQ

See *Pathology at a Glance* (**Breast carcinoma**).

Risk factors (each for ½ point):

Family history of breast malignancy, especially BRCA mutations

Age of menarche

Age of menopause (late menopause >50 years)

Age of first pregnancy (older increases risk)

Age

Gender (males may also develop breast malignancies)
Oral contraceptive pill
Smoking
Overweight

Fibroadenoma: benign neoplasm (½ point) seen in younger women. Mobile, smooth mass.

Intraductal papilloma: benign with sometimes bloody nipple discharge.

Paget disease of the breast: malignant (½ point). Eczematous appearing changes of the nipple. The Paget cells themselves are large, malignant cells but are indicative of an underlying breast carcinoma.

Fat necrosis: benign lump (½ point) that is often painful and seen in overweight/obese women with some trauma.

Ductal carcinoma: carcinomas by definition are malignant (½ point). If the basement membrane has not been penetrated the disease is known as ductal carcinoma *in situ*.

Answer 13: MCQ
See *Pathology at a Glance* (Tuberculosis).
(b) Tuberculosis is caused by *Mycobacterium tuberculosis* and is one of the most common infections worldwide. The majority of patients have latent, asymptomatic infections (d). Typical symptoms can be non-specific, including fevers, chills, night sweats and weight loss but you can also get haemoptysis (bloody sputum). The most common organ to be infected is the lung but TB can affect a wide variety of tissues including bone (Pott disease is infection of the spine, b), meningitis, gastrointestinal tract and genitourinary tract. Tuberculosis requires acid-fast staining (c), e.g. Ziehl–Neelsen, as gram staining is not useful. Treatment is for at least 6 months with multiple agents (a).

Answer 14: True/False
See *Pathology at a Glance* (T cells).
(a) **True**. Antigen-presenting cells (APCs) such as dendritic cells phagocytose pathogens and process them for presentation to CD4 T cells.
(b) **False**. Presentation by APCs to CD4 T cells is through MHC II whereas endogenous antigens (e.g. from intracellular viruses) are presented by cells on MHC I to CD8 T cells.
(c) **True**. CD4 T cells require interaction of CD28 to B7 (on APCs) for co-stimulation. Failure to provide this second stimulation results in anergy as the T cell assumes that it is a self-antigen, therefore preventing autoreactivity.
(d) **False**. B cells have B cell receptors, which include the immunoglobulin, that bind to antigens which are enocytosed and then presented on MHC II, like other APCs. Activated T cells then can stimulate the B cells to mature to plasma cells and make large quantities of antibodies.
(e) **True**. Although CD8 T cells recognise antigens presented on MHC I by any cell including APCs. However, they do not recognise antigens presented on MHC II by APCs.

Answer 15: MCQ
See *Pathology at a Glance* (Primary lung carcinoma).
(e) The history is consistent with a pulmonary malignancy. Smokers are at increased risk of bronchogenic carcinoma, especially squamous cell carcinoma and small cell carcinoma, both of which tend to be centrally located. Squamous cell carcinoma is associated with

PTHrP (parathyroid hormone-related peptide) secretion that can cause hypercalcaemia with a low PTH. Small cell carcinoma is associated with ADH (antidiuretic hormone) secretion and therefore high urine osmolality (b), and ACTH secretion (d). The symptoms of (c) are consistent with serotonin secretion from a carcinoma. Mesothelioma, a pleural malignancy (a), is rare, associated with asbestosis and has very poor prognosis.

Answer 16: True/False
See *Pathology at a Glance* (Viral hepatitis).
(a) **False**. Hepatitis A is an acute infection that is transmitted via the faecal–oral route and blood transfusion or sexual activity. Patients are not chronic carriers.
(b) **False**. Hepatitis B-vaccinated individuals are hepatitis B surface antibody positive but core antibody negative. If hepatitis B surface antigen was positive then an active infection would have been present, and the presence of hepatitis B surface antibody provides immunity. Hepatitis B is transmitted through sexual contact, exposure to contaminated needles and blood products, and vertical transmission from mother to fetus. Patients can become chronically infected and are at increased risk of cirrhosis and hepatocellular carcinoma.
(c) **True**. Hepatitis D only infects in the presence of hepatitis B. Co-infection or superinfection increases progression to hepatocellular carcinoma and cirrhosis.
(d) **True**. During this period, the body is clearing the surface antigen and developing a surface antibody response. However, these patients have already developed a core antibody response and therefore serological testing for hepatitis B needs to include this.
(e) **True**. Not all hepatitis B cases produce the e antigen. Clearance of the e antigen and demonstration of the antibody decrease viral load.

Answer 17: MCQ
See *Physiology at a Glance*, 3rd edn (Control of acid–base status).
(a) The kidney is essential in the maintenance of acid–base balance and potassium excretion. It is responsible for bicarbonate reabsorption primarily in the proximal nephron and excretion of acid primarily in the distal nephron. Failure of this process leads to metabolic acidosis (b). This is compensated for by hyperventilation and therefore decrease in pCO_2 (c).

Answer 18: True/False
See *Pathology at a Glance* (Assorted haematological conditions).
(a) **False**. Anaemia caused by vitamin B_{12} (cobalamin) and folate deficiency classically demonstrates megaloblasts in the bone marrow and hypersegmented neutrophils seen on peripheral blood smear.
(b) **True**. These two enzymes are involved in the metabolism of homocysteine and methylmalonyl-CoA. Therefore, in B_{12} deficiency serum homocysteine and serum and urine methylmalonic acid are elevated. An outdated test for vitamin B_{12} deficiency is the Schilling test.
(c) **False**. Vitamin B_{12} absorption requires binding to intrinsic factor and occurs in the ileum. Therefore, vitamin B_{12} deficiency is seen in Crohn disease in which terminal ileum inflammation is common.

(d) **False**. Neurological symptoms as described are seen in vitamin B$_{12}$ deficiency. Subacute degeneration of the spinal cord affects the lateral and dorsal columns and is associated with demyelination.

(e) **True**. Folic acid supplements are used in pregnancy to reduce the risk of neural tube defects, e.g. spina bifida, anencephaly.

Answer 19: MCQ

See *Pathology at a Glance* (**Acute and chronic pancreatitis**).

(a) The patient has pancreatitis, an acute inflammatory condition of the pancreas, that is potentially fatal. The two major causes are alcohol and gallstones (a) and together they account for three quarters of all cases. Other causes are remembered by the acronym GET SMASHED (gallstone, ethanol, trauma, steroids, mumps, autoimmune disease, scorpion bites, hypercalcaemia/hypertriglyceridaemia, ERCP, drugs).

Answer 20: MCQ

See *Medical Pharmacology at a Glance*, **7th edn**.

(c) Many antibiotics are teratogenic including tetracyclines, aminoglycosides, chloramphenicol NS sulphonamides, but amoxicillin is safe. Alcohol is the leading cause of congenital malformations in the Western world. Consequences include mental retardation, cardiac defects, facial defects and limb abnormalities. Warfarin should be replaced with heparin during pregnancy. Paracetamol and opiates are safe in pregnancy. NSAIDs are not teratogenic but can cause persistent ductus arteriosus, especially in the third trimester.

Answer 21: SAQ

See *Pathology at a Glance* (**Congenital heart disease**).
Shunts
Foramen ovale: shunting of most of the blood reaching the right atrium into the left atrium, thereby skipping the pulmonary circulation.

Ductus arteriosus: shunt between the pulmonary artery and aorta. Blood pumped into the pulmonary artery is shunted to the aorta and then into the rest of the fetal body.

Ductus venosus: shunt from the umbilical vein into the inferior vena cava, bypassing the liver. Therefore oxygenated blood from the placenta in the umbilical vein reaches the inferior vena cava.

Congenital cardiac defects
Tetralogy of Fallot: pulmonary stenosis, right ventricular hypertrophy, over-riding aorta, ventricular septal defect.

Total anomalous pulmonary venous return: pulmonary veins drain into the systemic venous circulation.

Transposition of the great vessels: can produce various combinations but in all, the major great vessels (pulmonary artery, pulmonary vein, aorta, superior vena cava and/or inferior vena cava) are misplaced. For example, right heart pumping into the aorta.

Truncus arteriosus: failure of the truncus arteriosus to split into the pulmonary artery and aorta.

Ventricular septal defect, atrial septal defect and patent ductus arteriosus are all causes of left-to-right shunt. However, over time this can become right-to-left shunt as the right heart hypertrophies. Known as Eisenmenger syndrome.

Answer 22: MCQ

See *Pathology at a Glance* (**Bronchiectasis**).

(a) The clinical features are classic for primary ciliary dyskinesia (also called Kartagener syndrome). It is characterised by ciliary immotility, which affects multiple organ systems: It causes bronchiectasis in the respiratory tract, infertility due to fallopian tube dysfuction and sperm immotility. Ciliary immotility also affects embryogenesis leading to situs inversus. Chediak–Higashi syndrome is due to a microtubule polymerisation defect (b), an immunodeficiency syndrome. (c) is seen in hereditary spherocytosis, (d) in respiratory distress syndrome in neonates, and (e) in cystic fibrosis.

Answer 23: SAQ

See *Pathology at a Glance* (**Miscellaneous non-neoplastic osteoarticular pathology**).

Calcitriol or 1,25-dihydroxycholecalciferol is the activated form of vitamin D$_3$. Vitamin D$_3$ is first hydroxylated in the liver by 25-hydroxylase and secondly at the kidneys by 1α-hydroxylase in a tightly regulated fashion (1). Deficiency in calcitriol leads to hypocalcaemia (2). Hyperphosphataemia occurs due to reduced phosphate excretion (3). Both these changes stimulate parathyroid hormone secretion and therefore secondary hyperparathyroidism (4). The bone suffers from a mineralisation defect and patients develop renal osteodystrophy (5).

Answer 24: EMQ

See *Pathology at a Glance* (**Genetic disease**) and *Medical Genetics at a Glance*, **3rd edn**.

(1) **B**. The presentation is consistent with familial hypercholesterolaemia. It is caused by a mutation in the LDL receptor, leading to very high levels of circulating LDL cholesterol. This is in turn predisposes to early-onset atherosclerotic disease and homozygotes and has a poor prognosis. On examination, tendon xanthomas, xanthelasmas and corneal arcus may be found.

(2) **G**. Marfan syndrome is a connective tissue disease. Fibrillin is a protein found in the extracellular matrix and is essential in the formation of elastic fibres. Aortic dissection may occur due to cystic medial necrosis. Other features seen include pectus excavatum, mitral valve prolapse, aortic regurgitation and high-arched palate.

(3) **C**. Neurofibromatosis type 1 is caused by a mutation of the neurofibromin gene located on chromosome 17. More than six café-au-lait spots is included in the diagnostic criteria for NF1. Other features include freckling in the axilla, optic glioma, iris hamartomas (called Lisch nodules) and phaeochromocytomas. NF2 is caused by a mutation on chromosome 22 and is characterised by bilateral acoustic neuromas.

(4) **D**. Huntington disease is caused by a trinucleotide repeat expansion of CAG in the Huntingtin gene on chromosome 4. The disease demonstrates anticipation, i.e. it presents earlier in subsequent generations. Other trinucleotide repeat disorders include fragile X syndrome (CGG), myotonic dystrophy (CTG) and Friedreich ataxia (GAA).

(5) **A**. Adult polycystic kidney diseases is an autosomal dominant disorder (infantile disease is due to a autosomal recessive

disorder), associated with berry aneurysms and therefore subarachnoid haemorrhages, hepatic cysts and mitral valve prolapse.

Answer 25: MCQ

See *Pathology at a Glance* (**Parathyroid gland pathology**).
(b) Multiple endocrine neoplasia type I (Wermer syndrome) is associated with gastric ulcers caused by a pancreatic neoplasm (Zollinger–Ellison syndrome). MEN I is associated with pituitary and parathyroid tumours (3 Ps). MEN II is associated with parathyroid tumour, phaeochromocytoma and medullary carcinoma of the thyroid. MEN III (also called IIb) is associated with phaeochromocytoma, medullar carcinoma of the thyroid and mucosal neuromas. Neurofibromas are seen in neurofibromatosis, which is also associated with phaeochromocytoma development.

Answer 26: SAQ

See *Pathology at a Glance* (**Ulcerative colitis and Crohn's disease**).
Location: ulcerative colitis is limited to the colon usually with rectal involvement. Crohn can affect any part of the gastrointestinal tract from the mouth to the anus, with the rectum usually spared. The terminal ileum is commonly involved (and may lead to B_{12} deficiency).

Macroscopic: Crohn – cobblestoning, fat wrapping; UC – mucosal pseudopolyps, mucosal inflammation, enlarging shallow ulcers.

Disease distribution: UC produces continuous colonic lesions. Crohn has patches of inflammation (skip lesions).

Depth of inflammation: UC – mucosal and submucosal. Crohn – transmural inflammation.

Histology: Crohn's – non-caseating granulomas. UC – crypt abscesses, no granulomas, ulcerations.

Complications: UC – colorectal carcinoma, toxic megacolon, colonic perforation, stenosis. Crohn – perianal disease, fistulas (e.g. colovesical, colovaginal), abscess formation, colorectal carcinoma less common, B_{12} and other nutritional deficiencies.

Answer 27: MCQ

See *Pathology at a Glance* (**Systemic vasculitis**).
(b) The condition described is temporal arteritis (giant cell arteritis). It requires urgent treatment with high-dose steroids to prevent visual loss due to ophthalmic artery occlusion. Polymyalgia rheumatica causes pain of the proximal muscles and should also be treated with steroids. Fibromyalgia is a chronic pain disorder (c). Coronary artery aneurysms are associated with Kawasaki disease and should be treated with aspirin.

Answer 28: MCQ

See *Pathology at a Glance* (**Sarcoidosis and syphilis**).
(b) Syphilis transmitted to the fetus from the mother can cause a wide variety of abnormalities, including Hutchinson's teeth (incisor abnormality), facial deformities, sensorineural deafness, palate defect and sabre shins. The presentation of a painless chancre is primary syphilis and can progress to secondary and tertiary syphilis. Treatment is with penicillin. *Treponema pallidum*, the spirochaete that causes syphilis, is not visualised with gram staining but instead requires dark-field microscopy or fluorescent antibody staining.

Answer 29: True/False

See *Pathology at a Glance* (**Pneumonia**).
(a) **True**. This question requires you to know firstly that *Streptococcus pneumoniae* is the most common cause of lobar pneumonia and secondly that *S. pneumoniae* are gram-positive diplococci. Other bacterial causes include *Haemophilus influenzae, Mycoplasma pneumoniae, Chlamydia pneumoniae, Legionella pneumophila* and *Staphylococcus aureus*.
(b) **True**. Cystic fibrosis leads to bronchiectasis and CF patients are at higher risk for pseudomonas. They therefore need adequate coverage for pseudomonas which includes third-generation ticarcillin or piperacillin, cefepime or ceftazidime, aminoglycosides and carbapenems, among others. Penicillin, amoxicillin, ampicillin, first- and second-generation cephalosporins and macrolides do not adequately cover pseudomonas. Other pulmonary infections include *Haemophilus influenzae, Staphylococcus aureus* and aspergillus.
(c) **False**. A CD4 count below 200 cells/mm³ indicates AIDS in a HIV-infected individual. Although AIDS patients may have *Staphylococcus aureus* pneumonia, the most concerning cause is for *Pneumocystis jirovecii* pneumonia. Treatment is with trimethoprim-sulfamethoxazole (co-trimoxazole).
(d) **True**. *Legionella pneumophila* are well treated with macrolides and quinolones, with azithromycin and levofloxacin, respectively, being the preferred choices.
(e) **False**. The case describes mycobacterium tuberculosis rather than *Mycoplasma pneumoniae* infection. *M. tuberculosis* requires oxygen and therefore prefers the upper lobes. Gram staining will not detect the bacteria, which requires specific acid-fast staining, e.g. Ziehl–Neelsen stain.

Answer 30: MCQ

See *Pathology at a Glance* (**Paediatric tumours**).
(a) A neuroblastoma is a tumour arising from the sympathetic nervous system. It is made up of small blue round cells and may form Homer–Wright rosettes. A nephroblastoma is a paediatric renal malignant tumour arising before 5 years of age. It is associated with Wilms tumour genes (WT1 and WT2) found on chromosome 11.

11 Neuroscience exam 1

Questions

Question 1: True/False

Following head injury, a patient is diagnosed clinically with dominant parietal lobe damage. Which features would allow such a diagnosis?

(a) Inability to calculate
(b) Disinhibition
(c) Non-fluent aphasia
(d) Inability to show the examiner how to cut bread
(e) Inability to name the fingers as thumb, index, middle, ring and little

Question 2: MCQ

A 75-year-old man has an amputation of his pinna secondary to skin cancer. Which of the following abilities will be most affected by this loss?

(a) Horizontal localisation
(b) Vertical localisation
(c) Balance
(d) Very high frequency sound perception
(e) Very low frequency sound perception

Question 3: MCQ

A 76-year-old man suffers a neurodegenerative condition and subsequently dies. Postmortem investigations show the affected cells (Figure 11.1). An arrow marks the affected cell type.

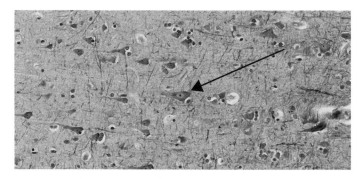

Figure 11.1 Histological image of the brain. © Regents of the University of Michigan, reproduced with permission. http://141.214.65.171/M2%20Pathology/Neuro/NormalNP004_20X.svs/view.apml.

(a) Astrocyte
(b) Microglial cell
(c) Oligodendrocyte
(d) Purkinje cell
(e) Pyramidal cell

Question 4: EMQ

A patient presents with Wallenberg syndrome, a medullary stroke syndrome. Its clinical signs and symptoms are outlined below. Please choose the correct anatomical correlation in Figure 11.2 for each of the symptoms of the syndrome.

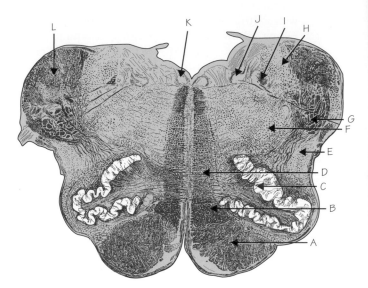

Figure 11.2 Coronal brain section.

(1) Ataxia
(2) Vertigo and vomiting
(3) Loss of pain and temperature sensation in the face
(4) Hoarseness
(5) Loss of pain and temperature sensation in the arms and legs

Question 5: SAQ (5 points)

A patient comes to your clinic complaining of low mood. What are the physical symptoms seen in depression that you should ask about?

Question 6: MCQ

A patient with right-sided homonymous hemianopia is admitted to a study. Although he is left completely blind following a resection of his left occipital lobe, he still responds to movement and light on the right. How is this explained?

(a) The autonomic nervous system, via the ciliary ganglion, conveys some visual information to the brainstem.
(b) The intact occipital lobe also receives some limited input from the opposite visual field.
(c) The lateral geniculate nucleus on the left projects to areas involved in the processing of visual information other than V1.
(d) The visual cortex receives visual input from both eyes.
(e) His vision relies on brainstem reflexes such as those that control pupillary sphincters.

Question 7: MCQ

A 67-year-old smoker is diagnosed with lung cancer. He also complains of weakness that is worst in the mornings and is found to have Lambert–Eaton myasthenic syndrome. The weakness in this syndrome is the consequence of an antibody against presynaptic calcium channels. This results in impairment of transmission at the neuromuscular junction. Which *one* statement about the actions of calcium in synaptic transmission is true?

(a) Presynaptic calcium concentrations do not affect the amplitude of the miniature endplate potential.
(b) Calcium binds to SNAP-25 to cause vesicle fusion.
(c) Calcium is released via ligand-gated calcium channels.
(d) Calcium causes vesicle release by binding to calmodulin kinase (CaMK).
(e) Calcium is necessary but not sufficient to cause synaptic transmission.

Question 8: MCQ

You assess the development of an 18-month-old child. Appropriate for her age, the child still has difficulty judging the distance of things she wants to pick up. What provides the cerebellum with the error message that allows for correction of the movement?

(a) Climbing fibre
(b) Mossy fibre
(c) Parallel fibre
(d) Deep cerebellar nuclei
(e) Purkinje cell

Question 9: EMQ

A Amygdala
B Cingulate gyrus
C Hippocampus
D Hypothalamus
E Mammillary body
F Medial prefrontal cortex
G Nucleus accumbens
H Parahippocampal gyrus
I Reticular formation
J Suprachiasmatic nucleus

For each scenario below, choose the correct answer from the list above.

(1) You are seeing a patient who has difficulties with recognising fearful stimuli and recognising facial expressions of fear. Which structure has been damaged in the subject?
(2) Three cavers are trapped underground without watches. They continue to sleep when tired and find the exit early on the third day. To their surprise it is morning outside, as expected. Which structure in the brain has allowed them to maintain a day-night cycle?
(3) 24-year-old man suffers head injury secondary to a traffic accident. While on intensive care, he is noted to be profoundly hypothermic. The hypothermia is resistant to treatment and he subsequently dies. The autopsy may find damage in which structure?
(4) You are looking after a patient with a long-standing heroin addiction who is asking for surgical treatment. Which area, involved in reward-guided learning and addiction, may be a potential target for inhibition by deep brain stimulation?
(5) A chronic alcoholic is admitted to a nursing home because he is no longer able to look after himself. He has a poor memory of events in his life, is forgetful and readily makes up stories to answer questions. Which of the above structures has classically been associated with this syndrome?

Question 10: True/False

When a person emerges from the dark into a sunlit space, initially everything appears white but within seconds to minutes vision returns to 'normal'. What are the mechanisms by which the eye can adapt to large variations in light intensity?

(a) Phosphorylation
(b) Pigment synthesis
(c) Calcium influx
(d) Pupillary constriction
(e) A two-receptor system

Question 11: SAQ (5 points)

You are looking at a postmortem spinal cord section of a sailor (Figure 11.3). It is noted that he was bedbound and confused prior to dying. What is the name of the involved anatomical structure? What symptoms does this lesion cause? What is the name of the condition and probable underlying aetiology?

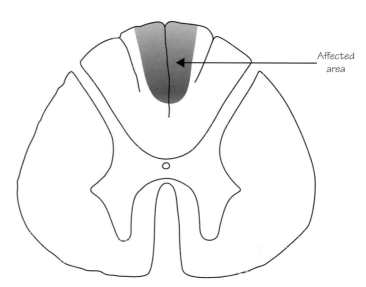

Affected area

Figure 11.3 Transverse section of the spinal cord showing the affected region.

Question 12: MCQ

You start a patient on haloperidol for an acute psychotic episode. Which of the following side-effects can occur?

(a) Akathisia (restlessness)
(b) Acute dystonia
(c) Parkinsonism
(d) Tardive dyskinesia
(e) All of the above

Question 13: EMQ

A BDNF
B Cell adhesion molecules
C Ephrins
D Neuregulin1 (Nrg1)
E Neurexin
F Neuroligin
G Netrins
H NGF
I NogoA

J Protocadherin
K Retinoic acid
L Sonic hedgehog

For each of the questions below, choose the most appropriate answer from the list above.

(1) Which secreted molecule helps neurons such as the corticospinal tract neurons to cross the midline? Knockout of the gene disrupts the development of axon pathways that cross the midline in experimental animals.
(2) Which morphogen is secreted from the notochord and floorplate of the developing spinal cord, which is important in establishing the identity of neurons in the ventral spinal cord? A mutation in the gene may result in holoprosencephaly – a failure of the brain to develop two hemispheres.
(3) This protein supports the outgrowth and survival of sympathetic neurons.
(4) These molecules provide gradients of inhibitory signals in the brain. This is best studied in the frog tectum where these molecules help to guide retinal axons to the correct part of the tectum.
(5) This molecule regulates synapse formation in humans. Its polymorphisms are associated with schizophrenia.

Question 14: MCQ

A patient with epilepsy and memory problems has an MRI scan, which shows hippocampal atrophy. Which of the following will be impaired?
(a) Declarative memory acquisition
(b) Declarative memory storage
(c) Non-declarative memory acquisition
(d) Non-declarative memory storage
(e) All of the above

Question 15: MCQ

You are trying to sleep on a night train but despite having your eyes closed, you notice when the train comes to a quick halt. How many balance organs do humans have?
(a) 3
(b) 4
(c) 6
(d) 8
(e) 10

Question 16: True/False

A patient suffers from a chronic demyelinating neuropathy. How does loss of myelin affect the patient's neurophysiology?
(a) It predominantly affects C fibres.
(b) It results in decrease of the amplitude on nerve conduction studies.
(c) It increases the capacitance of affected fibres.
(d) It reduces the velocity of conduction of fibres of all diameters.
(e) It can result in a block in conduction.

Question 17: MCQ

A medical student is spending day and night in the library prior to his final exams. This is an example of which reinforcement schedule?

(a) Continuous reinforcement schedule
(b) Fixed interval schedule
(c) Fixed ratio schedule
(d) Variable interval schedule
(e) Variable ratio schedule

Question 18: EMQ

A Photoreceptor
B On-centre bipolar cell
C Off-centre bipolar cell
D Amacrine cell
E Horizontal cell
F M-type ganglion cell
G P-type ganglion cell

For each of the questions below, choose the most appropriate answer from the list above.

(1) A doctor looks through the eye using an ophthalmoscope. Which cell layer is furthest from the observer?
(2) You observe a blue house against the background of the sea. Which cells synapse onto photoreceptors to effectively increase the contrast of the image seen?
(3) An experimental animal loses the ability to detect stimuli that are brighter than the background but retains the ability to see stimuli that are darker than the background. Which cell type has been pharmacologically inactivated?
(4) A forester looks at a footprint. Which cell will fire most action potentials with information about the shape of the footprint?
(5) You record from a cell in the retina which hyperpolarises in response to glutamate. What is the most likely cell type in question?

Question 19: MCQ

Following a stroke, a patient asks whether his nerve cells will regenerate. You reply that there is a limited possibility for adult nerve cell production in the following area:
(a) amygdala
(b) basal ganglia
(c) cortex
(d) hippocampus
(e) spinal cord

Question 20: SAQ (5 points)

You are standing 100 metres from a child who is 1 metre tall. What is the angle in degrees subtended by the image of the object and its size on your retina if you assume that your eye has a diameter of 17 mm?

Question 21: MCQ

A patient suffers an upper quadrantanopia following a stroke. What is the location of the stroke?
(a) Frontal lobe
(b) Temporal lobe
(c) Parietal lobe
(d) Occipital lobe
(e) Cerebellum

Question 22: True/False

A 43-year-old patient is admitted for electroconvulsive therapy (ECT). Which statements about ECT are true?

(a) Renal failure and raised creatine kinase are possible side-effects.
(b) Patients may experience anterograde amnesia.
(c) Patients may experience retrograde amnesia.
(d) Patients should be referred for ECT if there are life-threatening features of depression such as refusal of food.
(e) ECT can work after the first session.

Question 23: SAQ (5 points)
Name five areas of the hypothalamus and their functions.

Question 24: MCQ
A patient attends your otolaryngology (ENT) clinic complaining of hearing loss. The Rinne test is positive in both ears (i.e. normal) and Weber's test lateralises to the right. What pathology can explain the above findings?
(a) Left ear wax
(b) Right ear cholesteatoma
(c) Left ear drum perforation
(d) Left acoustic neuroma
(c) Right acoustic neuroma

Question 25: MCQ
You are investigating long-term potentiation. Which area on the light micrograph (Figure 11.4) receives input from the Schaffer collaterals and is the most investigated area of LTP?

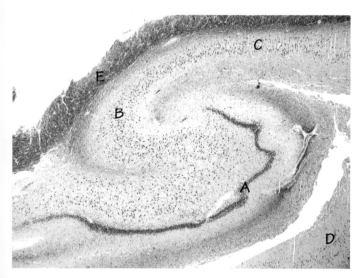

Figure 11.4 Sagittal brain slice. Reproduced courtesy of Dr Olaf Ansorge.

Question 26: True/False
'See no evil, hear no evil' ... feel no evil. Which of the following features do the senses of vision, hearing and touch share?
(a) All three senses have an input into the superior colliculus.
(b) All three sensory pathways synapse in the thalamus.
(c) The primary cortical areas retain an organisation that maintains the topography of its neuronal input.
(d) The receptors for all three senses hyperpolarise in response to stimulation.
(e) Changes in the physical environment are transmitted by amplitude-coded electrical signals.

Question 27: EMQ
A Agranulocytosis
B Anaemia
C Ataxia
D Bradycardia
E ECG abnormalities and arrhythmias
F Hypertensive crisis
G Parkinsonism
H Rash
I Respiratory depression

For each of the questions below, choose the most appropriate answer from the list above.
(1) You see a 65-year-old patient with a third seizure in 2 months. You decide to start him on lamotrigine. Which side-effect, which can be life-threatening, will you mention to the patient?
(2) You see a 43-year-old woman with depression who has taken a large overdose of a tricyclic antidepressant. What is the main reason for admission for observation?
(3) A 13-year-old girl has taken all her mother's diazepam. What will be the main focus of your examination and inpatient monitoring?
(4) You start a patient suffering from depression on phenelzine, a monoamine oxidase (MAO) inhibitor. You warn them not to eat aged cheeses and fermented foods because of a risk of which side-effect?
(5) A 25-year-old patient has failed multiple antipsychotic medications and has been a psychiatric inpatient for more than 6 months. He is started on clozapine, which requires monitoring for which severe side-effect?

Question 28: MCQ
A drug representative hands you the following prospectus. What information can you infer from Figure 11.5? Select *one* statement only.

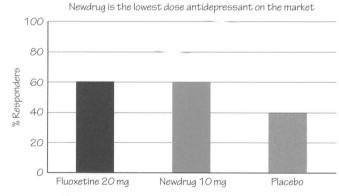

Figure 11.5 Graph showing the percentage of patients responding to fluoxetine, newdrug and a placebo.

(a) *Newdrug* has fewer side-effects.
(b) *Newdrug* is a selective serotonin reuptake inhibitor.
(c) *Newdrug* has similar efficacy to fluoxetine.
(d) *Newdrug* has a higher affinity for its target.
(e) If treatment with *newdrug* fails, fluoxetine will not be of benefit.

Question 29: SAQ (5 points)

Figure 11.6 shows a cross-sectional image of a sural nerve. What is the imaging technique used to obtain the image? Label the diagram.

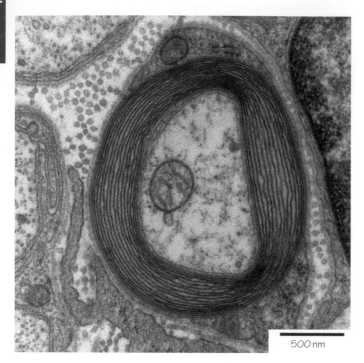

500 nm

Figure 11.6 Cross-sectional image of a sural nerve. Reproduced under the Creative Commons Licence from Trinity College, Hartford, Conneticut, USA.

Question 30: MCQ

An art gallery visitor looks at a painting. Which of the following structures is involved in the perception of colour?

(a) M-type ganglion cell
(b) Koniocellular LGN layer
(c) Interblob
(d) Area V5
(e) Area MT

Answers to Exam 1

Answer 1: True/False

See *Neuroanatomy and Neuroscience at a Glance*, 4th edn (Association cortices: the posterior parietal and prefrontal cortex).

The parietal lobe is involved in the organisation of sensory percepts into complex concepts. Lesions of the parietal lobe may cause apraxia – the inability to carry out tasks despite seemingly normal power. Dominant parietal lobe lesions may cause further symptoms that are collectively known as Gerstmann syndrome if they occur together (although they rarely do): acalculia, finger agnosia, agraphia and right–left disorientation.

(a) **True**. This is known as acalculia.
(b) **False**. This is a feature of frontal lobe damage.
(c) **False**. Broca's area is found in the inferior frontal cortex.
(d) **True**. This is known as apraxia.
(e) **True**. This is known as finger agnosia.

Answer 2: MCQ

See *Neuroanatomy and Neuroscience at a Glance*, 4th edn (Auditory system II).

(b) The pinna serves the collection and amplification of sounds that reach the inner ear, and it particularly enhances midrange frequencies that correspond to the bandwidth of vocalisation (d,c) rather than frequencies at the extremes of hearing. It also has a function in the localisation of sound, and allows us to distinguish particularly the vertical orientation of sound (b). The vestibular apparatus will not be affected by alteration in the external ear (c).

Answer 3: MCQ

See *Neuroanatomy and Neuroscience at a Glance*, 4th edn (Cells of the nervous system I and II).

(e) The characteristic triangular shape of pyramidal cells (hence their name), their irregular soma and the presence of a large apical dendrite allow for their easy identification on histology slides (e).

Answer 4: EMQ

See *Neuroanatomy and Neuroscience at a Glance*, 4th edn (Anatomy of the brainstem and Cerebrovascular disease).

The Wallenberg syndrome is also known as the *lateral* medullary syndrome. It is characterised by infarction of the dorsolateral medulla; it is thus unsurprising that all the symptoms will have anatomical correlates that are clustered in that region.

(1) **L**. Ataxia arises through infarction of the inferior cerebellar peduncles.
(2) **H**. Infarction of the vestibular nuclei causes symptoms of vertigo and vomiting.
(3) **G**. This is the location of the spinal nucleus of the trigeminal nerve. The long spinal nucleus reaches down into the medulla and is responsible for pain and temperature sensation.
(4) **I**. This is the nucleus ambiguus which contains the motor fibres innervating the laryngeal and pharyngeal muscles that travel in cranial nerves IX and X.
(5) **E**. The spinothalamic tract is found laterally in the medulla. It carries pain and temperature sensation.

Answer 5: SAQ

See *Neuroanatomy and Neuroscience at a Glance*, 4th edn (Neurochemical disorders I: affective disorders).

Sleep disturbance (early morning wakening or oversleeping)
    Loss of energy
    Loss of concentration
    Change in appetite or weight (overeating and anorexia)
    Psychomotor agitation or retardation

Answer 6: MCQ

See *Neuroanatomy and Neuroscience at a Glance*, 4th edn (Visual system III and Consciousness and theory of mind).

(c) 'Blindsight', the ability to see some stimuli despite complete blindness on conventional testing, is a fascinating phenomenon that occurs in a minority of patients with lesions of the visual cortex, usually following occipital strokes. Various theories have been put forward for this phenomenon, including vision through residual V1 cortex and alternative pathways via the superior colliculus. In macaque monkeys with blindsight, destruction of the lateral geniculate nucleus abolishes that skill, indicating that it is a key component in pathways that allow vision in the absence of V1 cortex (c). The autonomic nervous system does not convey complex visual information, even though it controls pupillary diameter (a). There is good evidence that the information from one hemifield travels only to the opposite occipital lobe (b). The fact that this information comes from the same hemifield of both eyes cannot explain blindsight (d). Brainstem reflexes cannot explain blindsight, which is a complex cortical phenomenon (e).

Answer 7: MCQ

See *Medical Sciences at a Glance* (Neuromuscular transmission) and *Neuroanatomy and Neuroscience at a Glance*, 4th edn (Neuromuscular junction and synapses).

(a) A rise in presynaptic calcium concentration is both necessary (i.e. no transmission without calcium) and sufficient (i.e. no other ions are required) to cause synaptic transmission in humans (e). The arrival of the action potential causes the opening of voltage-gated calcium channels (c). Calcium causes immediate fusion of vesicles by binding directly to synaptotagmin (b), a vesicular protein. Calcium only exerts *some* (much slower) actions by activating calmodulin-dependent kinase (d). Variations in calcium levels, like the reduction seen in Lambert–Eaton myasthenic syndrome, change the frequency but not the amplitude of a single miniature endplate potential. The amplitude depends on the amount of neurotransmitter in a single vesicle, which remains unchanged (a). However, endplate potentials themselves, which are a compound of *miniature* endplate potentials, *are* reduced in Lambert–Eaton syndrome.

Answer 8: MCQ

See *Neuroanatomy and Neuroscience at a Glance*, 4th edn (Cerebellum).

(a) The cerebellar circuit is a feedback control system. The key output cell is the Purkinje cell (e). Mossy fibres that relay a large amount of information from the cortex provide the input (b).

Climbing fibres originate in the superior olive and provide modulation and correction of movement. Their input has a modifying effect on the parallel fibre input into the Purkinje cell (a).

Answer 9: EMQ

See *Neuroanatomy and Neuroscience at a Glance*, 4th edn (Limbic system and Emotion, motivation and drug addiction).

(1) **A**. Conditioned fear responses localise to the amygdala as functional MRI imaging and studies in mice have shown. The best-known human subject is SM, who has bilateral damage to her amygdala secondary to a genetic condition. She has difficulty recognising fear in other persons and does not report the emotion of fear.

(2) **J**. The suprachiasmatic nucleus is situated in the anterior part of the hypothalamus, and is responsible for controlling circadian rhythms, which are generated by a gene expression cycle. It controls other hypothalamic nuclei and the pineal glands, modulating the production of hormones, including cortisol and melatonin.

(3) **D**. Thermoregulation is one of the key functions of the hypothalamus, and hypo- and hyperthermia have both been reported following damage to it.

(4) **G**. Surgical treatment of addiction is experimental and rarely done in modern times. The nucleus accumbens is a natural target for deep brain stimulation, also being known as the 'pleasure centre' of the brain. It receives dopaminergic inputs from the ventral tegmental area which can be greatly amplified during drug taking.

(5) **E**. The syndrome described above, characterised by anterograde and retrograde amnesia as well as confabulation and emotional blunting, is Korsakoff syndrome. It is caused by thiamine deficiency and although it has been observed secondary to starvation, its most common cause is alcoholism. Neuroanatomically, this syndrome has classically been linked with mammillary body atrophy. However, the profound memory problems correlate best with thalamic injury. The mammillary body has been implicated in visuospatial memory.

Answer 10: True/False

See *Neuroanatomy and Neuroscience at a Glance*, 4th edn (Sensory transduction).

It is a general truth that physiological amplification cascades have an inbuilt off-switch. This is particularly important for the eye, which works with intensities of light that differ by a factor of 10^6.

(a) **True**. Inactivation of receptors by phosphorylation is a common element of signalling cascades that is also found in the retina. Once activated, rhodopsin becomes a target for phosphorylation by opsin kinase, which renders it susceptible to inactivation by another protein called arrestin.

(b) **False**. Light adaptation does not involve pigment synthesis.

(c) **True**. This is probably the major pathway that desensitises cones and allows hyperpolarised photoreceptors to return to the usual depolarised membrane potential. In the dark, calcium enters photoreceptors through the same channels as sodium. Calcium inhibits guanylate cyclase (produced in darkness). On light exposure, the ion channels close, reducing the Ca^{2+} concentration in the cell and thereby releasing cGMP production. Over time, this counteracts the decrease in cGMP

caused by light stimulation and returns the membrane to its original depolarised state, thereby resetting the set point.

(d) **True**. Pupillary constriction plays a role but can only account for a small reduction in retinal stimulation.

(e) **True**. The availability of two types of receptors specialised for light (cones) and low light (rods) conditions respectively greatly increases the range.

Answer 11: SAQ

See *Neuroanatomy and Neuroscience at a Glance*, 4th edn (Clinical disorders of the sensory systems).

The image in Figure 11.3 shows dorsal column pathology, specifically affecting the fasciculus gracilis (1). This structure carries fine touch and proprioceptive information from the lower limbs (2), but the patient's pain and temperature sensation would remain intact (3). Degeneration of the dorsal columns, particularly the fasciculus gracilis, is known as tabes dorsalis (4) and was seen frequently in tertiary syphilis prior to the widespread availability of antibiotics (5).

Answer 12: MCQ

See *Neuroanatomy and Neuroscience at a Glance*, 4th edn (Neurochemical disorders II).

(e) Haloperidol, like most antipsychotics, is a D2 receptor antagonist and therefore can cause a range of extrapyramidal side-effects which include akathisa, dystonia within days, parkinsonism usually within weeks to months and tardive dyskinesia within months to years.

Answer 13: EMQ

See *Neuroanatomy and Neuroscience at a Glance*, 4th edn (Neural plasticity and neurotrophic factors I).

(1) **G**. Netrins are a group of families that are chemoattractants. They are localised to the floorplate of the neural tube and attract and help axons that need to cross the midline.

(2) **K**. Sonic hedgehog is a morphogen expressed both in the notochord as well as the floorplate. Among many other functions, it is important in ventrodorsal patterning of the spinal cord as well as neural tube closure.

(3) **H**. Neurotrophins, such as BDNF, NGF and NT-3/4, are specialised signalling molecules that are homologous in amino acid sequence and have specificity to support a particular type of neuron. They are secreted by neuronal targets. The specificities of these molecules are best established in the PNS where NGF supports predominantly sympathetic fibres, BDNF supports Merkel cell discs and NT-3 supports muscle spindles.

(4) **C**. Ephrins are important axon guidance molecules that provide repellent and attractive signals to growing axons. They have been best studied in the frog tectum where retinal axons find their target in two-dimensional space using gradients of different ephrin signalling.

(5) **D**. Neuregulin is a transmembrane protein that is released following cleavage of its extracytoplasmic portion. The soluble part then binds to neuronal receptors and regulates synapse formation by recruiting transmembrane proteins.

Answer 14: MCQ

See *Neuroanatomy and Neuroscience at a Glance*, 4th edn (Memory).

(a) Patients with hippocampal atrophy as seen in severe temporal lobe epilepsy and early Alzheimer disease have intact declarative

Table 11.1 The areas of the brain involved in acquiring and storing different types of memory.

	Acquisition	Storage
Declarative memory	Hippocampus	Cerebral cortex
Non-declarative memory (implicit memory)	Unknown	Basal ganglia, cerebellum, premotor cortex

memories of things past but have difficulty with forming new declarative memories and have poor short-term memory.

Non-declarative memories are the unconsciously stored information on how to perform a certain task, such as how to reach for a cup; these are linked to the basal ganglia and cerebellum amongst others (Table 11.1).

Answer 15: MCQ

See *Neuroanatomy and Neuroscience at a Glance*, 4th edn (Vestibular system).

(e) In each ear there are five balance organs: three semicircular canals, the utricle and the saccule. This makes a total of 10 balance organs.

Answer 16: True/False

See *Neuroanatomy and Neuroscience at a Glance*, 4th edn (Nerve conduction and synaptic integration).

(a) **False**. C fibres are unmyelinated and are thus least affected by demyelinating polyneuropathies.

(b) **False**. In demyelinating neuropathies, the myelin sheath is lost, without a loss of axons. This results in slower conduction but normal amplitude.

(c) **True**. Myelination decreases the capacitance of the nerve fibre. The membrane capacitance is the ability of the axonal wall to store energy, like a battery. Because this process requires time, it slows down conduction. An increase in the capacitance results in slower conduction overall.

(d) **False**. Myelination is only beneficial for larger fibres; smaller fibres actually are slowed by myelin, which is the reason why C fibres are unmyelinated.

(e) **True**. Conduction block is a feature of demyelinating disease. It results in decreased conductance between the nodes of Ranvier, and the impulses may not reach the node and thus extinguish the action potential. High temperatures exacerbate this.

Answer 17: MCQ

(b) Exams occur at fixed intervals and result in a steeply rising curve of response. After an exam, there is usually an interval during which there is no response but response increases exponentially as the next deadline approaches (b). A continuous reinforcement schedule would involve daily mini-exams (a), a variable interval schedule would involve unannounced exams scattered throughout the year (d). Fixed ratio schedules would reward for every five pieces of work produced (c), whereas variable ratio schedules would unpredictably yield a reward after a piece of work was

handed in, e.g. praise in front of all other students on excellent completion of an assignment (e).

Answer 18: EMQ

See *Neuroanatomy and Neuroscience at a Glance*, 4th edn (Visual system I).

(1) **A**. Rather counterintuitively, the retina is arranged so that the photoreceptors sit on the basal membrane furthest away from the incident light, with all other retinal cells, nerves, veins and arteries on top of them.

(2) **E**. The only cells that synapse onto photoreceptors are horizontal cells. Horizontal cells lay the foundations for the centre-surround organisation of the optic pathway which remains important even in the visual cortex. The centre-surround organisation effectively allows us to see borders and edges more clearly, i.e. increases contrast.

(3) **B**. Bipolar cells are responsible for detecting changes in luminance and come in two different types. On-centre bipolar cells increase their discharge to luminance increments, whereas off-centre bipolar cells increase their discharge in response to luminance decrements.

(4) **G**. The only cells that fire action potentials in the retina are ganglion cells. The P-type cells (parvocellular, midget ganglion cells) are specialised in detecting shapes and structures, and to some extent also colour.

(5) **C**. Hyperpolarisation (inhibition) by glutamate is an unusual property of some bipolar retinal cells, as glutamate is usually excitatory. This is mediated by a G-protein-coupled receptor mechanism similar to the one in the photoreceptor: activation of the G-protein cascade results in stimulation of phosphodiesterase and fall in cAMP concentrations that ultimately result in the closure of potassium channels. This mechanism is found in off-centre bipolar cells.

Answer 19: MCQ

See *Neuroanatomy and Neuroscience at a Glance*, 4th edn (Neural plasticity and neurotrophic factors II).

(d) There is evidence of limited adult neurogenesis in the hippocampus (d). It is unknown if these new cells make functioning connections, and the overall purpose of this phenomenon is unknown. The only other site in the brain where neurogenesis occurs in humans is the olfactory bulb, not mentioned in this question. There is now good evidence against adult neurogenesis in the human cortex (c) as evidenced by carbon-14 labelling experiments. This means that our stroke patient will not be able to benefit from this mechanism; he can, however, be assured that there is good evidence for plasticity in the adult brain and for good outcomes from rehabilitation.

Answer 20: SAQ

Firstly, you need to calculate the angle α subtended by the image (1). This is calculated using basic trigonometry as $\tan \alpha = \frac{x}{d}$ (2, 3), where d is the distance of the object and x is its height, thus in our case this is 0.57°.

You can use simple proportionality to calculate the size of the retinal image (4): $\frac{size\ of\ image}{diameter\ of\ retina} = \frac{x}{d}$, thus the size of the image will be 1/100 of the diameter of the retina, i.e. 170 μm (5). This corresponds to 85 cones.

Answer 21: MCQ

See *Neuroanatomy and Neuroscience at a Glance*, 4th edn (Visual system II).

(b) The optic radiation splits in half on its way from the lateral geniculate nucleus to the striate cortex. The fibres from the upper half of the visual field (the lower half of the retina) traverse the temporal lobe (b, also known as Meyer's loop), while the lower half of the visual field passes through the parietal lobe (c). There are no projections of the visual pathway in the frontal lobe and cerebellum (a,e), while occipital lobe lesions cause hemianopia, as the upper and lower radiations are reunited there (d).

Answer 22: True/False

(a) **False**. ECT is done under anaesthesia and muscle relaxation is routinely administered.

(b) **True**. Patients commonly suffer anterograde amnesia. This is transient.

(c) **True**. Patients suffer declarative memory loss with ECT. This appears to be greater for impersonal information than autobiographical information.

(d) **True**. The main indications for ECT are life-threatening depression or severe treatment-resistant depression.

(e) **True**. ECT is one of the few treatments with immediate effects (others include stimulant therapy) and has the most evidence for efficacy and best safety profile of these treatments.

Answer 23: SAQ

See *Neuroanatomy and Neuroscience at a Glance*, 4th edn (Hypothalamus).

Suprachiasmatic nucleus: controls circadian rhythm
  Lateral nucleus: controls hunger and thirst
  Arcuate nucleus: controls hormone release from pituitary
  Medial preoptic area: controls sexual behaviour (in animals)
  Ventromedial nucleus: satiety centre, controls reflex behaviour such as responses to hunger and thirst

Answer 24: MCQ

(d) The fact that the Rinne test is positive in both ears indicates that the hearing loss is sensorineural (d, e) rather than conductive (a-c). In sensorineural hearing loss Weber's test lateralises to the healthy ear, in our case the right. This is the opposite of conductive hearing loss where the diseased ear has an intact but oversensitive hearing apparatus and thus Weber's test localises to the diseased ear.

Answer 25: MCQ

See *Neuroanatomy and Neuroscience at a Glance*, 4th edn (Limbic system and long-term potentiation).

(c) Long-term potentiation occurs in multiple regions, but currently the region that is most investigated is CA1 (c) which receives Shaffer collaterals that originate in CA3 (b).

Answer 26: True/False

See *Neuroanatomy and Neuroscience at a Glance*, 4th edn (Sensory systems: an overview and Visual system II).

(a) **True**. The superior colliculus receives visual input arranged in a topographical map of visual space and is supplemented by sensory and visual stimuli that are arranged in a similar fashion. The sensory input is closely integrated with a topographical map of eye movements that underlies saccadic responses to new stimuli.

(b) **True**. Both major sensory pathways and the auditory and visual pathways synapse in thalamic nuclei, which relay the information to the cortex. The thalamus has a poorly understood but probably important role in stimulus processing.

(c) **True**. All three sensory cortices have an organisational structure that is organised similarly to its input. The somatosensory cortex is organised somatotopically, as illustrated by the sensory homunculus, the visual cortex is organised retinotopically and the auditory cortex has a tonotopic arrangement.

(d) **False**. While photoreceptors hyperpolarise in response to light, they are unique in this property. Pain fibres, mechanoreceptors and hair cells depolarise in response to stimulation.

(e) **False**. As action potentials are all-or-nothing, all signals are frequency coded. Amplitude coding would not work because the action potential amplitude decreases with the distance travelled, and is regenerated along the axon.

Answer 27: EMQ

See *Neuroanatomy and Neuroscience at a Glance*, 4th edn (Neurochemical disorders I and II and Neurophysiological disorders).

(1) **H**. Lamotrigine is one of the more commonly prescribed antiepileptics. It is a preferred drug in the elderly because of its lack of interactions. Rashes are the most common side-effect, affecting 10% of patients. It is important to discontinue the drug immediately when a rash occurs.

(2) **E**. Tricyclic antidepressants are 'dirty' drugs acting on multiple receptors. They have a wide range of side-effects including glaucoma, urinary retention, constipation and delirium.

(3) **I**. Respiratory depression from benzodiazepines is not uncommon in the hospital setting, and causes include self-harm and overmedication. It is important to monitor the respiratory rate when giving these drugs, especially intravenously.

(4) **F**. Non-selective MAO inhibitors interact with tyramine-containing foods such as aged cheese and fermented food products. MAO inhibition prevents the breakdown of tyramine, which then displaces noradrenaline from the vesicles into the synapse, causing a noradrenergic crisis.

(e) **A**. Clozapine is tightly monitored because of a significant risk of agranulocytosis – loss of neutrophils that makes patients susceptible to sepsis.

Answer 28: MCQ

See *Medical Sciences at a Glance* (Basic mechanisms of drug action) and *Neuroanatomy and Neuroscience at a Glance*, 4th edn (Neurochemical disorders I).

(c) Prospectuses and lectures from drug companies often present data in such a way as to create subconscious associations which may be invalid. The fact that the doses of the two drugs are different has no bearing on any parameter that would interest the clinician. What this prospectus says is that *newdrug* is just as good as fluoxetine. It does not tell us about the mechanism of the drug (b), or of its affinity to its receptor (d). It also does not tell us about side-effects (a): the dose here is of no value as side-effects depend on a number of other variables. Finally, all antidepressants have very limited efficacy and there is a chance that a second-line antidepressant will work in 25% of cases – although both drugs work in 60% of patients, this does not mean they work on the *same* 60%.

Answer 29: SAQ

See *Neuroanatomy and Neuroscience at a Glance*, **4th edn (Cells of the nervous system II)**.
Figure 11.7 is a cross-sectional transmission electron micrograph (TEM) of a peripheral nerve, with all the major structures labelled.

Answer 30: MCQ

See *Neuroanatomy and Neuroscience at a Glance*, **4th edn (Visual system III)**.
(b) Colour perception is processed in parallel with other information streams in the visual pathway. Distinct structures are involved in its processing. In the retina, it is predominantly non-M non-P type ganglion cells and some P-type ganglion cells (a), in the lateral geniculate nucleus it is the interlaminar areas, also known as the

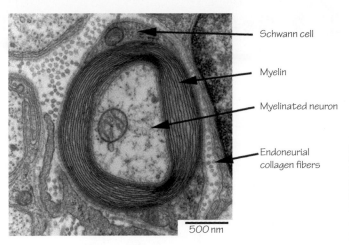

Schwann cell

Myelin

Myelinated neuron

Endoneurial collagen fibers

500 nm

Figure 11.7 Labelled cross-sectional transmission electron micrograph (TEM) of a sural nerve. Reproduced under the Creative Commons Licence from Trinity College, Hartford, Conneticut, USA.

koniocellular layers, that respond to colours most intensively (b). These feed directly to the cytochrome oxidase blobs in layer 2 (c). Area V5 and MT are concerned with the onward processing of movement beyond the visual cortex (d,e).

12 Neuroscience exam 2

Questions

Question 1: EMQ

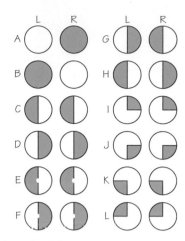

Figure 12.1 Various visual field defects.

For each of the scenarios below, choose the most appropriate visual defect from Figure 12.1.
(1) A 27-year-old woman is diagnosed with multiple sclerosis following inflammation of her left optic nerve.
(2) A 56-year-old publican has a complete left-sided posterior circulation stroke. What would his visual defect look like?
(3) A 43-year-old patient is diagnosed with an aneurysm following a visual field defect secondary to involvement of the right optic tract. What is the visual field defect corresponding to this presentation?
(4) A 24-year-old woman presents with secondary amenorrhoea and tirednesss. She is found to have a pituitary macroadenoma. What visual field defect would you expect?
(5) A 24-year-old woman undergoes a right temporal lobectomy for her intractable and medication-resistant epilepsy. What kind of visual field defect should she be warned about prior to surgery?

Question 2: MCQ

A 55-year-old patient with migraine attends your clinic. His episodes are not frequent but very debilitating. You therefore choose to start a reliever. Which of his following co-morbidities will stop you from prescribing a 5-HT1A receptor agonist such as sumatriptan?
(a) Gastritis
(b) Previous myocardial infarction
(c) Benign prostatic hyperplasia
(d) Chronic kidney disease
(e) Epilepsy

Question 3: MCQ

A patient in a sleep study is found sleepwalking. What is his EEG most likely to show?

(a) Stage I sleep
(b) Stage II sleep
(c) Stage IV sleep
(d) REM sleep
(e) Awake EEG

Question 4: True/False

A 64-year-old man has a history of tremor and rigidity. He is bradykinetic. He is diagnosed with idiopathic Parkinson disease. Which of the following treatment options may be useful in this condition?
(a) Selective inhibition of the globus pallidus internus by deep brain stimulation.
(b) Selective destruction of the globus pallidus externus.
(c) Inhibition of the subthalamic nucleus by deep brain stimulation.
(d) Inhibition of the substantia nigra by deep brain stimulation.
(e) Inhibition of the thalamus by deep brain stimulation to reduce tremor (excess movement).

Question 5: MCQ

When a photon reaches its receptor molecule in the human eye, a signalling cascade is activated. Which of the following best describes this cascade?
(a) Ligand-gated ion channel
(b) Calcium-mediated calcium release
(c) Tyrosine kinase receptor
(d) G-protein-coupled receptor
(e) Transcriptional activation

Question 6: EMQ

A Extraocular muscles
B Cranial nerve III
C Cranial nerve IV
D Cranial nerve VI
E Parapontine reticular formation
F Nucleus raphe interpositus
G Median longitudinal fasciculus
H Rostral interstitial nucleus of the medial longitudinal fasciculus
I Superior colliculus
J Frontal eye fields
K Cerebellum
L Vestibular nucleus

For each of the scenarios below, select the structure that has most probably been affected.
(1) A 25 year-old woman presents with a hoarse voice, general weakness in her arms and drooping of her eyelids. She complains of double vision, especially on looking up. On examination, there is fatigable weakness of eye movements.
(2) A 24-year-old woman with morbid obesity presents with a gradual-onset headache that is worse in the mornings. She

also complains of double vision. On examination, she is unable to abduct the left and the right eye.

(3) A 30-year-old woman who has a history of multiple sclerosis complains of new-onset double vision. On examination, she can look to the right but on looking to the left, the right eye does not adduct and the right eye abducts with nystagmus.

(4) A 67-year-old woman with signs of parkinsonism is diagnosed with progressive supranuclear palsy. She is unable to look up or down. What is the cause of this gaze palsy?

(5) A patient with epilepsy undergoes video telemetry. During a typical fit, he is observed to assume a fencing posture. During the seizure the patient fixes his gaze to the right. What structure has been involved by the seizure?

Question 7: SAQ (5 points)

A 77-year-old patient suffers from atrial fibrillation, high blood pressure and anaemia and uses a stick to walk. He is on ramipril, furosemide, digoxin and warfarin. He also has a steroid inhaler and tiotropium for his COPD. During his last hospital admission he was started on phenytoin for seizures. He now asks about side-effects of the medication because he doesn't feel right. What are the side-effects in relation to the history of this patient?

Question 8: True/False

A person gets chilli onto broken skin and experiences pain. What is true about the active ingredient in hot peppers and its receptor?

(a) It can be used in treatment of chronic pain.
(b) The active ingredient in hot peppers acts intracellularly.
(c) The receptor is also sensitive to changes in extracellular pH.
(d) The receptor is a 7-transmembrane domain receptor.
(e) The receptor is expressed only on unmyelinated fibres.

Question 9: MCQ

After a period of abstinence, a 55-year-old man with alcoholism attends a party at which he sees a corkscrew. After a few minutes he goes to a nearby off-licence and begins binge drinking. How is the corkscrew best described?

(a) Conditioned response
(b) Conditioned stimulus
(c) Unconditioned response
(d) Unconditioned stimulus
(e) None of the above

Question 10: SAQ (5 points)

A patient with renal failure has hyperkalaemia. His serum potassium is 8 mmol/L. Compared to normal serum potassium, how does this influence the resting potential and excitability of nerve fibres?

Question 11: MCQ

A 56-year-old man comes to your clinic following a recent admission for stroke. His wife reports that he has difficulty recognising and responding to things to the left of him. The patient himself is adamant that he does not have any difficulties. During examination, when asked to pick up a glass of water standing left of him, he denies its existence. Where does his stroke localise?

(a) Left frontal lobe
(b) Left occipital lobe
(c) Left parietal lobe

(d) Right occipital lobe
(e) Right parietal lobe

Question 12: MCQ

The mechanism of long-term potentiation and depression underlies the acquisition of memory in mammals. Which *one* of the following statements is true about long-term potentiation (LTP) and depression (LTD)?

(a) It is only found in the hippocampus.
(b) LTP is specific for the postsynaptic cell; once established, the cell will be activated.
(c) LTP and LTD occur at the same synapse.
(d) The molecular mechanism underlying associativity is based on the properties of the AMPA receptor.
(e) LTP can persist for hours.

Question 13: MCQ

A patient suffers a thalamic stroke with involvement of the lateral geniculate nucleus (LGN). Which *one* of the following is true of this structure?

(a) It receives the majority of its input from retinal ganglion cells.
(b) It is retinotopically organised.
(c) It integrates input from both eyes.
(d) A patient with a stroke involving the LGN will suffer monocular blindness.
(e) 10% of its output goes to the midbrain tectum.

Question 14: SAQ (5 points)

You follow up a 75-year-old patient over some years. He initially presents with rigidity and bradykinesia. You soon notice unsteadiness and find that he has nystagmus and past-pointing. He also complains of difficulty with passing urine and has postural hypotension. Finally when examining him at a later stage, you find a positive Babinski response and brisk reflexes. For each of the signs and symptoms, identify the name of the clinical presentation and the anatomical location. What is the name of the condition that the patient suffers from?

Question 15: MCQ

A young man takes an antihistamine for his hay fever. After taking it, he becomes drowsy and has to lie down for a nap. Which pathway interfered with his wakefulness?

(a) Cholinergic nuclei
(b) Raphe nuclei
(c) Locus coeruleus
(d) Tuberomammillary nucleus of the hypothalamus
(e) Nucleus accumbens

Question 16: MCQ

You hold a mobile phone in your hand and notice it starts vibrating at a low frequency of 30 Hz. Which skin receptor helps you notice this so that you can pick up the call?

(a) Meissner's corpuscle
(b) Merkel cells
(c) Pacinian corpuscle
(d) Ruffini endings
(e) All of the above

Question 17: EMQ

A ATP
B Endorphin
C Dopamine
D GABA
E Glutamate
F Glycine
G Histamine
H Noradrenaline
I Substance P
J Serotonin

For each scenario below, choose the correct answer from the list above.

(1) A 25-year-old man with spinal cord trauma undergoes experimental treatment to reduce the tonic inhibition in his spinal cord. Modulation of which neurotransmitter would selectively achieve this?
(2) Which neurotransmitter may be involved in the pathobiology of schizophrenia as evidenced by the fact that phencyclidine (PCP) causes both negative and positive psychotic symptoms?
(3) A 22-year-old man who suffers from panic attacks takes his daily diazepam. Diazepam relieves anxiety by enhancing the action of which neurotransmitter?
(4) A 66-year-old woman is prescribed an antipsychotic for challenging behaviour secondary to her newly diagnosed dementia. A week later her family bring her to the emergency department with falls. She has marked rigidity on examination. Inhibition of which neurotransmitter has caused this?
(5) Patients successfully treated for depression were enrolled in an experiment. They were given a tryptophan-depleted diet. Within 24h, their symptoms of depression returned. This experiment provided further evidence for a role of which neurotransmitter in depression?

Question 18: SAQ (5 points)

A 24-year-old woman takes valproate for epilepsy. She attends her GP because of a positive pregnancy test at home. What developmental abnormality is more common with valproate and many other antiepileptic medications? At which stage of development does this occur? Can anything be done to prevent it?

Question 19: MCQ

During a ward round, one of the doctors says: 'This patient has an extrapyramidal disorder'. This means…
(a) the patient clinically has a disorder of the basal ganglia
(b) the patient is feigning their symptoms
(c) the patient has a clinical diagnosis of Parkinson disease
(d) the patient has a psychiatric disorder
(e) the patient has an illness that does not involve the corticospinal tract.

Question 20: True/False

Which of the following statements about conditioned responses in drug use and withdrawal is true?
(a) The police find an intravenous drug user (IVDU) injecting a dose of heroin. They take him to the police station. Immediately after entering the cell, he gets a withdrawal reaction, which is an example of operant conditioning.
(b) A man arrives intoxicated at the pharmacy requesting his methadone. The pharmacist refuses to give it to him. This is an example of negative reinforcement.
(c) An ex-IVDU is overcome by cravings when seeing his old girlfriend with whom he injected. This is a conditioned response.
(d) An intravenous drug user never misses an appointment at the methadone clinic because he loathes the withdrawal effects so much. This is an example of classical conditioning.
(e) A drug user injects his drug; this action is known as the unconditioned stimulus.

Question 21: MCQ

Human nerves use active conduction to transmit action potentials. How does it differ from passive conduction?
(a) It is faster.
(b) It allows for a more truthful representation of information.
(c) It is always all-or-nothing.
(d) It is always saltatory.
(e) It is not found in myelinated fibres.

Question 22: MCQ

While performing a neurological examination, you assess a patient with a large fibre demyelinating neuropathy. His power is normal but his reflexes are absent. Which fibres have been affected by the neuropathy to cause the absent reflexes?
(a) α-Motor neuron
(b) Ib Golgi tendon organ afferents
(c) γ-Motor neuron
(d) Ia muscle spindle afferents
(e) II muscle spindle afferents

Question 23: EMQ

A Pinna
B Stapes
C Helicotrema
D Dorsal cochlear nucleus
E Ventral cochlear nucleus
F Medial superior olive
G Lateral superior olive
H Inferior colliculus
I Superior colliculus
J Medial geniculate complex
K Lateral geniculate nucleus
L Primary auditory cortex

For each of the scenarios below, choose the most appropriate answer from the list above.

(1) Which part of the auditory system is crucial for the localisation of someone shouting above you?
(2) Which part of the auditory system allows you to know where the high-frequency singing of a bird is coming from?
(3) Which part of the auditory system localises the low-frequency noise of a car approaching?
(4) On hearing a loud noise, your eyes immediately fixate on the point in space where the sound originated. Which structure is crucial for the integration of auditory and visual information?
(5) You see a patient with monoaural deafness due to acoustic neuroma. Which structure makes it possible for this man to still be able to localise sounds?

Question 24: True/False

You prescribe amitriptyline for neuropathic pain. The patient asks about side-effects. Which of the following side-effects will you mention?

(a) Dizzy turns via α-adrenergic blockade
(b) Dry mouth via antimuscarinic effects
(c) Palpitations via β-agonism
(d) Sedation via H_1-receptor blockade
(e) Inability to empty the bladder via α-adrenergic agonist action

Question 25: MCQ

You are seeing a 20-year-old patient with a severe depressive episode that started after her grandmother died. When faced with a difficult situation in life, what factors can predispose a person to developing depression?

(a) External attribution
(b) Stable attribution
(c) Specific attribution
(d) None of the above
(e) All of the above

Question 26: MCQ

A 32-year-old woman with an Arnold–Chiari malformation presents with neurological symptoms due to a syrinx at the level of C7. Which function will be affected first due to enlargement of the spinal canal?

(a) Axial musculature
(b) Appendicular musculature
(c) Sweating
(d) Temperature sensation
(e) Vibration sensation

Question 27: True/False

You are seeing a teenage patient with a depressive episode. Which of the following statements is true about the treatment of depression?

(a) Medications are more efficacious than psychotherapy.
(b) Most teenagers on selective serotonin reuptake inhibitors (SSRIs) experience suicidal ideation.
(c) Most antidepressants have similar efficacy.
(d) Most psychotherapies have similar efficacy.
(e) If the patient requires rapid treatment of depression, atypical antipsychotics injected under the skin (depot) are the treatment of choice.

Question 28: EMQ

For each of the scenarios choose the most appropriate brain structure from the list in Figure 12.2.

(1) A 76-year-old woman presents with falls. You note marked past-pointing. Which structure is damaged?
(2) A 67-year-old woman presents with involuntary movements of her arms. Her father, who also had dementia, suffered from a similar condition in his later life. Which structure is probably involved?
(3) An 80-year-old man presents with weakness of his left arm. He has marked drooping of the face on the left. There are no sensory deficits. Which structure is involved?
(4) A 16-year-old boy presents with a history of headache that is worse in the mornings. On examination, he has loss of vertical

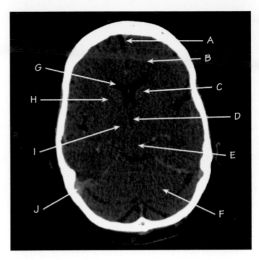

Figure 12.2 CT of the brain.

gaze and large pupils with a sluggish reaction to light. Which area is affected?

(5) A young man develops loss of consciousness after a stroke. Involvement of which structure in stroke may result in loss of consciousness?

Question 29: SAQ (5 points)

A worker is using a jackhammer when a heavy truck goes by. Both sounds have a sound pressure level of 100 decibels. What is the combined sound pressure level of these two sounds when added together? The worker wonders if the combined noise exceeds the legal limit of 130 decibels. (The reference sound pressure for calculation of decibels is $2*10^{-5} pascals$.)

Question 30: MCQ

You perform a voltage clamp experiment using a giant squid axon. Using the usual experimental set-up, you cause depolarisation by setting the voltage to obtain the result shown in Figure 12.3.

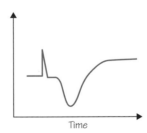

Figure 12.3 Action potential voltage trace.

(a) The y axis represents the voltage changes during an action potential.
(b) The initial spike is the excitatory postsynaptic potential.
(c) The initial downturn is due to an increase in potassium conductance.
(d) The graph represents the probability of opening of a sodium channel at a given time during the action potential.
(e) The cell remains depolarised throughout the experiment.

Answers to Exam 2

Answer 1 EMQ

See *Neuroanatomy and Neuroscience at a Glance*, **4th edn** (**Visual system II**).

Please note that visual fields are depicted as the patient sees them; thus, unlike most other diagrams and imaging modalities in medicine, right is right and left is left.

(1) **B.** An optic nerve lesion is prechiasmal, and will thus affect one eye only.

(2) **F.** This lesion is postchiasmal, and will thus affect the same hemifield of both eyes (homonymous hemianopia). In this case the posterior cerebral artery supplies the entire visual cortex – with the exception of some collateral circulation by the anterior circulation to the fovea, resulting in foveal sparing.

(3) **C.** The optic tract is the nerve bundle that connects the optic chiasm and the lateral geniculate nucleus. As the lesion is postchiasmal, you would expect a hemianopia as the presenting feature of a lesion. Unlike in scenario 2, you would not expect any foveal sparing.

(4) **H.** Pituitary tumours often present with visual field defects. As the pituitary is located immediately above the optic chiasm, it classically affects the central fibres of the chiasm that supply the nasal retina and therefore the temporal visual fields. The resulting defect is a bitemporal hemianopia.

(5) **I.** As part of the optic radiation passes through the temporal lobe, it is not surprising that 50–90% of patients undergoing temporal lobe resections have some visual impairment on examination following their surgery. The fibres travelling through the temporal lobe receive their input from the upper contralateral quadrant of the visual field and patients may experience a complete or partial upper quadrantanopia.

Answer 2 MCQ

See *Medical Sciences at a Glance* (**CNS disorder and treatments**) and *Neuroanatomy and Neuroscience at a Glance*, **4th edn** (**Main CNS neurotransmitters**).

(b) The use of 5-HT1 receptor agonists in migraine is explained by the vascular hypothesis of migraine. This assumes that dilation of the blood vessel underlies the headache and 5-HT1 agonists cause vasoconstriction. It is thus unsurprising that significant cerebral, coronary and peripheral vascular disease are contraindications to their use.

Answer 3: MCQ

See *Neuroanatomy and Neuroscience at a Glance*, **4th edn** (**Reticular formation and sleep**).

(c) Against common misconception, sleepwalking takes place during deep sleep, i.e. stages III and IV (c). It does not occur during REM sleep (d). Should the EEG show an awake rhythm, you can be sure the patient is not sleepwalking (e).

Answer 4: True/False

See *Neuroanatomy and Neuroscience at a Glance*, **4th edn** (**Basal ganglia and their treatment**).

The substantia nigra modulates two pathways of movement generation that originate in the striatum: it inhibits the indirect pathway,

which acts to stop movements, and activates the direct pathway, which decreases the tonic inhibition on the thalamus and thus allows movement. In Parkinson disease this balance is disturbed, and the lack of modulation by the substantia nigra (pars compacta) results in underactivity of the direct pathway and overactivity of the indirect pathway, both of which increase the tonic inhibition of the thalamus and thus stop movement.

In reality, the use of deep brain stimulation is more complex than described in this question. For example, globus pallidus internus stimulation can be effective in both chorea and parkinsonism, and stimulation of globus pallidus externus has also been used to treat parkinsonism. Nevertheless, the modulation by deep brain stimulation is predominantly inhibitory and the question serves to illustrate the principles behind the basal ganglia circuit.

(a) **True.** Inhibition of the globus pallidus internus is a major target in deep brain stimulation for Parkinson disease. It tonically inhibits the thalamus, so its inhibition causes improvements in voluntary movements.

(b) **False.** Lesioning of the globus pallidus externus could exacerbate symptoms of Parkinson disease. As seen in Figure 12.4, its output is already diminished in Parkinson disease and further damage to it would cause further activation of the subthalamic nucleus and exacerbation of Parkinson symptoms. This has been shown in experiments on monkeys.

(c) **True.** The subthalamic nucleus is the second major target for deep brain stimulation in Parkinson disease. It is part of the indirect circuit and is overactive in parkinsonian patients due to loss of inhibition by the globus pallidus internus.

(d) **False.** The substantia nigra is never a target for deep brain stimulation. Inhibition of the substantia would exacerbate the symptoms. Its degeneration is the cause for Parkinson disease.

(e) **True.** Tremor is one of the most treatment-resistant features of Parkinson disease. Deep brain stimulation of the thalamus, specifically the ventral intermediate part, has had some encouraging results in tremor-predominant Parkinson disease.

Answer 5: MCQ

See *Neuroanatomy and Neuroscience at a Glance*, **4th edn** (**Sensory transduction**).

(d) The signalling system in human photoreceptors consists of a 7-transmembrane-receptor protein called rhodopsin, which serves as a photon sensor, and a G-protein called transducin. This system allows for amplification of the photon stimulus and is speedy.

Answer 6: EMQ

See *Neuroanatomy and Neuroscience at a Glance*, **4th edn** (**Eye movements**).

(1) **A.** The history of extraocular symptoms as well as the fatigable weakness are suggestive of myasthenia gravis. This is an autoimmune condition acting typically on the nicotinic acetylcholine receptors at the neuromuscular junction.

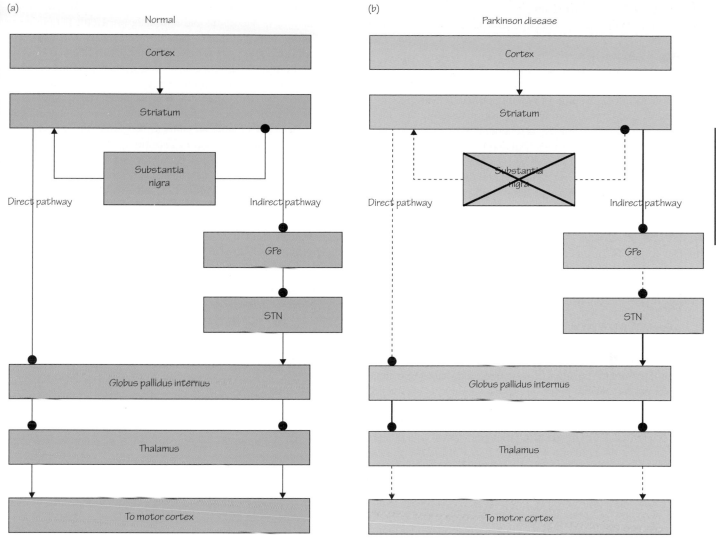

(a) Normal

(b) Parkinson disease

Figure 12.4 Pathways of movement generation in (a) normal and (b) patients with Parkinson disease.

(2) **D**. This is known as a 'false localising sign'. The history suggests a 'high pressure' headache, in this age group most likely due to idiopathic intracranial hypertension. Because cranial nerve VI has such a long course over the clivus, it is particularly susceptible to damage by raised intracranial hypertension. This can cause unilateral or bilateral VI nerve palsies resulting in inability to abduct the affected eye.

(3) **G**. The history of multiple sclerosis gives a hint – this condition is classically associated with intranuclear ophthalmoplegia. The clinical history does indeed fit this condition. It is due to a plaque involving the medial longitudinal fasciculus.

(4) **H**. The rostra interstitial nucleus of the medial longitudinal fasciculus receives inputs from the frontal eye fields and superior colliculus and projects to the oculomotor nuclei controlling vertical gaze and vertical saccades.

(5) **J**. The suggestion of a fencing posture localises the seizure to the frontal lobe, but even without this suggestion, gaze direction is controlled by the frontal eye fields. Stimulation of one frontal eye field produces eye movement in the contralateral direction, and this can be seen during epileptic seizures involving the frontal eye fields.

Answer 7: SAQ

See *Neuroanatomy and Neuroscience at a Glance*, 4th edn (Neuro-physiological disorders).

Phenytoin is still commonly used in clinical practice as it is found on most status epilepticus flowcharts. It is not the best choice and there are particular problems in the elderly who will be on many other medications also. In this case the following side-effects are likely to be of significance.

Can lower warfarin levels.

Can lower digoxin levels.

Ataxia and nystagmus causing difficulty with balance.

Peripheral neuropathy can also contribute to decreased mobility.

Can worsen anaemia through vitamin B_{12} deficiency.

Rashes are common and can be life threatening.

Sedation and drowsiness can increase risk of falls.

Answer 8: True/False

See *Neuroanatomy and Neuroscience at a Glance*, **4th edn (Pains systems II)**.

(a) **True**. Capsaicin is licensed for treatment of chronic pain; it works by desensitising pain receptors.

(b) **True**. The binding site for capsaicin is located intracellularly on the vanilloid receptor 1 (VR1). Capsaicin is hydrophobic, as evidenced by the fact that it dissolves in chilli oil.

(c) **True**. The VR1 receptor reacts to a number of stimuli other than capsacin, which include heat and low pH.

(d) **False**. The VR1 receptor is a non-selective cation channel.

(e) **False**. Pain fibres can be myelinated and unmyelinated. Myelinated pain fibres are of the Aδ subtype and are important in the immediate reaction to pain.

Answer 9: MCQ

(b) The corkscrew in this case is a conditioned stimulus (b). It is associated with the unconditioned stimulus of drinking alcohol (d) and the unconditioned response of alcohol intoxication (a). Craving is the conditioned response to the corkscrew (a).

Answer 10: SAQ

See *Neuroanatomy and Neuroscience at a Glance*, **4th edn (Resting membrane and action potential)**.

At rest, the membrane potential in nerve fibres is dependent predominantly on the equilibrium potential for potassium, as at rest the cell membrane is predominantly permeable to potassium (1). As the membrane is permeable predominantly to potassium at rest, the membrane potential can be estimated using the Nernst equation (2), which states that the equilibrium potential is $E = \frac{kT}{ze} \ln \frac{[K]_{out}}{[K]_{in}}$. This can be simplified to $E = 61 \log \frac{[K]_{out}}{[K]_{in}}$ at body temperature. For potassium at normal concentration the equilibrium constant is around −90 mV (assuming intracellular potassium is 120 mmol/L and the extracellular concentration is 4 mmol/L), and this becomes −70 mV in our patient with hyperkalaemia, thus resulting in a relative depolarisation (3). The relative depolarisation theoretically makes membranes more excitable, as it is easier to induce an action potential (4), but membrane excitability is decreased as the relative depolarisation causes sodium channels to remain in the inactivated form for longer (5).

Answer 11: MCQ

See *Neuroanatomy and Neuroscience at a Glance*, **4th edn (Association cortices)**.

(e) This is a classic description of left-side neglect. The features that distinguish this case from a left-sided hemianopia (right occipital lobe defect, d) is the fact that the patient denies the existence of the left side. Patients with occipital lobe defects are aware that there is part of their vision missing and will attempt to compensate for this. For patients with neglect, the left side simply does not exist. This particular patient has no insight into his neglect; patients with neglect can have insight into their condition but will remain clear that for them that part of the world simply does not exist.

Answer 12: MCQ

See *Medical Sciences at a Glance* **(Central nervous system function)** and *Neuroanatomy and Neuroscience at a Glance*, **4th edn (Limbic system and long-term potentiation)**.

(c) Long-term potentiation has been hypothesised to underlie the formation of memory in mammals and humans. It was initially discovered in the hippocampus but has since been observed in the cerebral cortex, cerebellum and amygdala (a). LTP/LTD are input specific, thus only the synapse that activated LTP/LTD becomes activated, allowing selectivity for given memories (b). LTP and LTD do occur at the same synapse and both result in calcium influx of different magnitudes that has opposite effects (c). Key to the initiation of LTP/LTD is the NMDA receptor (normally blocked by Mg^{2+} ions), which allows for calcium influx only when there is concomitant depolarisation by another stimulus at the same time; this requirement of temporal coincidence of two stimuli underlies the property of associativity that is key to LTP and memory (d). AMPA receptors are also present at the same synapse and result in depolarisation of the membrane but do not induce LTP and do not give rise to associativity. The calcium release triggers calcium-dependent kinase activation, which results in persistent changes at the synapse. Ultimately these changes result in altered gene transcription and protein synthesis, allowing the changes to last for more than 1 year (e).

Answer 13: MCQ

See *Medical Sciences at a Glance* **(The sensory system) and** *Neuroanatomy and Neuroscience at a Glance*, **4th edn (Visual system II)**.

(b) The lateral geniculate nucleus is not simply a relay station between the retina and the visual cortex. It receives 90% of the retinal output, while 10% of the retinofugal projection goes directly to the midbrain tectum, bypassing the LGN (e). Despite receiving the majority of the retinal output, this only makes up a minority of the LGN input, while 80% of its input comes from the visual cortex (a). Each LGN receives input from the same hemifield of both eyes, so the patient in the vignette will suffer a homonymous hemianopia rather than monocular blindness (d). The LGN keeps the inputs from both eyes separate rather than integrating them, so that LGN neurons will fire preferentially in response to stimuli in one eye – an example of parallel processing (c). Finally, the LGN is organised retinotopically like the whole of the visual pathway. This means that inputs that are adjacent to each other on the retina remain close to each other throughout the cortex.

Answer 14: SAQ

See *Neuroanatomy and Neuroscience at a Glance*, **4th edn (Clinical disorders of the motor system and Basal ganglia diseases and their treatment)**.

The patient is suffering from multiple systems atrophy, a rare condition sometimes called one of the 'Parkinson plus syndromes. It results in progressive degeneration of multiple motor systems, though not all have to be involved.

Rigidity and bradykinesia – parkinsonism – basal ganglia

Nystagmus and past-pointing – ataxia – cerebellum

Postural hypotension and urination difficulties – autonomic dysfunction – autonomic nervous system

Upgoing plantars and brisk reflexes – upper motor neuron damage – corticospinal tract

Answer 15: MCQ

See *Medical Sciences at a Glance* **(Central nervous system function)**.

(d) Histaminergic projections to the brain arise from the tuberomammillary nucleus of the hypothalamus and play a key role in mediation of wakefulness and arousal. They act directly via projections to the cortex and thalamus but also indirectly increase wakefulness via modulating cholinergic output.

Answer 16: MCQ

See *Medical Sciences at a Glance* (The sensory system) and *Neuroanatomy and Neuroscience at a Glance*, 4th edn.

(a) There are two types of rapidly adapting receptors in the human skin. Meissner's corpuscles convey their information via rapidly adapting I afferents and respond best to low frequencies (a). The rapidly adapting II afferents are attached to Pacinian corpuscles, which have very large receptive areas that best respond to frequencies 200–300 Hz (c). Merkel cells and the less well-characterised Ruffini organs are slowly adapting and play a role in fine tactile discrimination and perception of stretch and object motion respectively.

Answer 17: EMQ

See *Neuroanatomy and Neuroscience at a Glance*, 4th edn (Main CNS neurotransmitters and their function and Neurotransmitters, receptors and their pathways).

(1) **F**. The predominant inhibitory neurotransmitter in the cord is glycine. Experimental inhibition with strychnine, which is a competitive antagonist of glycine, has been attempted in the treatment of spasticity after spinal cord injury. It is highly toxic and poorly tolerated and thus not used in clinical practice.

(2) **E**. Glutamate is the main excitatory neurotransmitter in the brain and it acts on NMDA and AMPA receptors. The glutamate hypothesis is one of the major alternatives to the dopamine hypothesis in schizophrenia. One of the lines of evidence supporting this is the emergence of psychotic symptoms after the use of PCP, which is an NMDA receptor antagonist.

(3) **D**. GABA is an inhibitory neurotransmitter in the brain. Drugs acting on the GABA receptor have anxiolytic effects. Benzodiazepines act on the GABA receptors to increase the probability of its opening in response to GABA binding.

(4) **C**. Rigidity and postural instability (falls) are two of the major hallmarks of parkinsonism. Dopamine antagonism is one of the side-effects of antipsychotic medications. With a history of dementia and such a marked reaction to antipsychotic drugs, you may consider dementia with Lewy bodies in your differential.

(5) **J**. Tryptophan is a precursor for serotonin, which is implicated in the development of depression. The major evidence for serotonin comes from the action of serotonin reuptake inhibitors such as fluoxetine (Prozac). The experiment in this question results in *acute tryptophan depletion* and demonstrates that reduced serotonin is a cause and not just an effect of depression.

Answer 18: SAQ

See *Neuroanatomy and Neuroscience at a Glance*, 4th edn (Neurophysiological disorders).

Many antiepileptic medications (especially valproate) are associated with spina bifida, a congenital condition caused by incomplete fusion of the caudal neural tube. This often results in an incompletely fused vertebral column and sometimes bulging of the spinal cord from that defect. Neural tube fusion occurs at day 26 after fertilisation, and thus often before the mother is aware she is pregnant. Therefore, preconception planning is important for women with epilepsy: firstly, to select the most appropriate antiepileptic, and secondly, to start the patient on 5 mg of folic acid prior to conception, which has been shown to prevent neural tube defects.

Answer 19: MCQ

See *Neuroanatomy and Neuroscience at a Glance*, 4th edn (Spinal cord motor organisation: descending motor pathways).

(a) Kinnier Wilson (of Wilson disease) coined the term 'extrapyramidal' in the 1920s to clinically describe disorders of basal ganglia, recognising that they have distinct presentations from corticospinal tract disorders and cerebellar disorders (a). Although it most often means that the patient clinically has Parkinson disease, it can also be used to describe choreiform movement disorders including Huntington disease (c). The term is specifically reserved for basal ganglia disorders: cerebellar disorders, for example, although formally not involving the pyramids/corticospinal tract ,are never described this way (e).

Answer 20: True/False

(a) **False**. An induced withdrawal reaction that is associated with a place is most probably due to classical conditioning. The patient has no control over the conditioned stimulus: he is overcome by the withdrawal response associated with the conditioned stimulus of being in a room previously associated with withdrawal.

(b) **False**. This is an example of punishment, specifically negative punishment. The pharmacist is taking away a reward that the patient receives in a fixed interval conditioning regimen. An example of negative reinforcement is given in question (d).

(c) **True**. The association of drug taking with certain people and paraphernalia is thought to be due to classical conditioning.

(d) **False**. The drug user here makes a conscious choice of getting the methadone – this is a good example of operant conditioning with negative reinforcement, i.e. doing something in order to avoid negative consequences.

(e) **True**. Delivery of a drug is an unconditioned stimulus. Its delivery results in the unconditioned response. It is unconditioned because it does not depend on the development of an association.

Answer 21: MCQ

See *Neuroanatomy and Neuroscience at a Glance*, 4th edn (Nerve conduction and synaptic integration) and *Medical Sciences at a Glance* (Nervous conduction).

(c) To conduct over larger distance than a few millimetres, nerve fibres have adapted to regenerate the action potential along the length of the axon: this is called *active conduction*. This regeneration takes time, making it slower (a). Because regeneration results in amplification of the amplitude, this becomes meaningless and thus the signal becomes 'all-or-nothing' (c). Due to this, amplitude can no longer code for the intensity of the signal, and this has to be coded in other ways (frequency, spatial), losing some of the detail of the original signal (b). Active conduction *does* occur in myelinated fibres (e), where gaps exist in the myelin to allow for regeneration, resulting in saltatory conduction (jumping from gap to gap). Saltatory conduction is not found in unmyelinated fibres (d).

Answer 22: MCQ

See *Neuroanatomy and Neuroscience at a Glance*, 4th edn (Muscle spindle and lower motor neuron).

(d) The stretch reflex consists of an afferent limb (Ia afferents of the muscle spindle) and an efferent limb (α-motor neuron). In this case we know that this is a predominantly sensory neuropathy because power is normal. Ia afferents are among the largest sensory fibres and respond to a change of muscle spindle length and are commonly affected in large fibre sensory neuropathies (d). Type II spindle afferents fire predominantly at rest to indicate the overall length of the spindle (e), whereas Golgi tendon organs are activated when the muscle is contracted (b) and neither plays a role in the stretch reflex. As power is normal, we know that the efferent limb of the spinal reflex is intact (a).

Answer 23: EMQ

See *Neuroanatomy and Neuroscience at a Glance*, 4th edn (Auditory system II).

(1) **A**. The pinna provides the basis for vertical sound localisation by altering the sound reaching the eardrum: the pinna induces a 'notch' by silencing a particular frequency that depends on the elevation of the sound source.

(2) **F**. The medial superior olive receives input from both ears and probably functions as a coincidence detector. For low frequency sounds, it analyses the incident of the waveform to determine which ear receives an input first.

(3) **G**. The lateral superior olive distinguishes high-frequency sounds (above 3 kHz). It does so by comparing the amplitude or intensity of the sound reaching both ears.

(4) **I**. The superior colliculus receives retinotopically organised visual data and topographically organised auditory data and also contains closely paired motor pathways that are capable of initiating cascades.

(5) **A**. Contrary to what you may think, it is still possible to localise sounds with one ear only. The design of the pinna gives the ability to localise sound not only coming from above but also from other directions. This becomes important when other mechanisms fail.

Answer 24: True/False

See *Neuroanatomy and Neuroscience at a Glance*, 4th edn (Neuro-chemical disorders I).

(a) **True**. α-Adrenergic receptor antagonism is seen in tricyclic antidepressants. It results in orthostatic hypotension and reflex tachycardia.

(b) **True**. Tricyclics are powerful anticholinergics that can result in dry mouth, urinary retention, constipation and glaucoma.

(c) **False**. Palpitations can be caused by tricyclics as described in (a), or via their arrhythmogenic effects.

(d) **False**. Tricyclics cause central sedative effects by inhibiting histaminergic pathways.

(e) **False**. Tricyclic antidepressants can indeed cause retention, but do this via the anticholinergic actions described in (b). They have α-adrenoreceptor *antagonist* properties.

Answer 25: MCQ

(b) According to the attributional model of depression, *internal* ('it's my fault', a), *stable* ('I would have never managed', b) and *global* ('I'm not good enough', c) attribution of life events predisposes to the development of depression.

Answer 26: MCQ

See *Neuroanatomy and Neuroscience at a Glance*, 4th edn (Clinical disorders of the sensory system).

(d) To answer this question you need to visualise a cross-section of the spinal cord. The spinal canal is central and all long fibre tracts, including the corticospinal tract, spinothalamic tracts and dorsal columns, are all relatively distant from it. Slightly closer are the anterior, intermediate and posterior horns containing the cell bodies of the respective pathways. However, just anterior to the spinal canal is the anterior commisure, which contains the spinothalamic neurons that have entered the spinal cord at this level. Thus pinprick and temperature sensation *at the level of the syrinx* are lost first.

Answer 27: True/False

(a) **False**. Cognitive behavioural therapy is an effective treatment, especially in mild-to-moderate depression. However, antidepressants have also shown significant benefit in the treatment of depression but have a slow onset of action during which side-effects may be common.

(b) **False**. SSRIs have been linked with suicidal ideation in teenagers and should only be used in conjunction with psychotherapies. It is important to note that suicidal ideation occurred in 3% of patients on SSRIs compared with 2% of patients taking placebo. SSRIs are still the first-choice antidepressant in adolescents if required.

(c) **True**. Many antidepressant medications appear equally effective. There is some evidence that some newer antidepressants have fewer side-effects.

(d) **True**. For those psychotherapies with a similar amount of evidence such as intrapersonal psychotherapy, cognitive behavioural therapy and exercise therapy, it does not appear to matter which one is selected.

(e) **False**. Antidepressants usually take many weeks to work although beneficial effects may be seen in the first 2 weeks. If rapid response is required for severe suicidal ideation or catatonic depression, electroconvulsive therapy is the treatment of choice.

Answer 28: EMQ

See *Neuroanatomy and Neuroscience at a Glance*, 4th edn (Examination of the nervous system and Neuroradiological anatomy).

(1) **F**. Past-pointing is a specific cerebellar sign (in the absence of weakness).

(2) **C**. The condition described is Huntington disease. It is characterised by caudate atrophy.

(3) **H**. The description above is classic of a lacunar stroke involving the internal capsules: a hemisensory deficit without involvement of higher function.

(4) **E**. This is a description of Parinaud syndrome. In the age group described, it is most probably due to a pineal gland tumour. The tumour compresses the dorsal midbrain, which includes the superior colliculus and Edinger–Westphal nuclei. The oculomotor nuclei may also be involved, causing diplopia. Although multiple structures in Figure 12.2 are

involved with eye movements, vertical gaze palsies localise to the midbrain.

(5) **I**. Loss of consciousness is a rare symptom and presentation in stroke should make you think of another diagnosis such as a seizure or cardiac event. When it happens, it usually indicates involvement of both thalami.

Answer 29: SAQ

The decibel scale is logarithmic. Thus, a sound of pressure P can be expressed in decibels as follows: $dB = 20\log\frac{P}{2*10^{-5}}$ (1). You first divide the decibels by 20 and take the inverse log (2). You then multiply this by $2*10^{-5}$, which should give you the result 2 pascals (3). Adding the two tones together results in a total pressure of 4 pascals (4). Plugging this back into the formula gives a total pressure of 106 decibels, which is still within legal limits (5).

Answer 30: MCQ

(d) As suggested in the name of the experiment, the voltage is 'clamped' and set to a constant value, which results in the opening of voltage-gated channels and thus induces changes seen during an action potential (e). The only way to achieve constant voltage is by 'injecting' current through the electrode in the face of changing resistance during the action potential, and this is measured by the *y* axis (a,c). Measuring the current allows quantification of the current and thus the conductance of the membrane during an action potential. The initial spike is an artefact caused by the fact that the nerve is a capacitor (b).

Index